Dosage Calculations for Nursing Students

Master Dosage Calculations the Safe and Easy Way Without Formulas

Second Edition

AUTHORS:

Bradley J. Wojcik, PharmD

Chase Hassen

Disclaimer

Although the author and publisher have made every effort to ensure that the information in this book was correct at press time, the author and publisher do not assume and hereby disclaim any liability to any party for any loss, damage, or disruption caused by errors or omissions, whether such errors or omissions result from negligence, accident, or any other cause.

This book is not intended as a substitute for the medical advice of physicians. The reader should regularly consult a physician in matters relating to his/her health and particularly with respect to any symptoms that may require diagnosis or medical attention.

All rights reserved. No part of this publication may be reproduced, distributed, or transmitted in any form or by any means, including photocopying, recording, or other electronic or mechanical methods, without the prior written permission of the publisher, except in the case of brief quotations embodied in critical reviews and certain other noncommercial uses permitted by copyright law.

NCLEX®, NCLEX®-RN, and NCLEX®-PN are registered trademarks of the National Council of State Boards of Nursing, Inc. They hold no affiliation with this product.

Some images within this book are either royalty-free images, used under license from their respective copyright holders, or images that are in the public domain.

© Copyright 2019 by Chase Hassen & Bradley J Wojcik, PharmD. All rights reserved.

ISBN: 9781096128748

First, I want to give you this FREE gift...

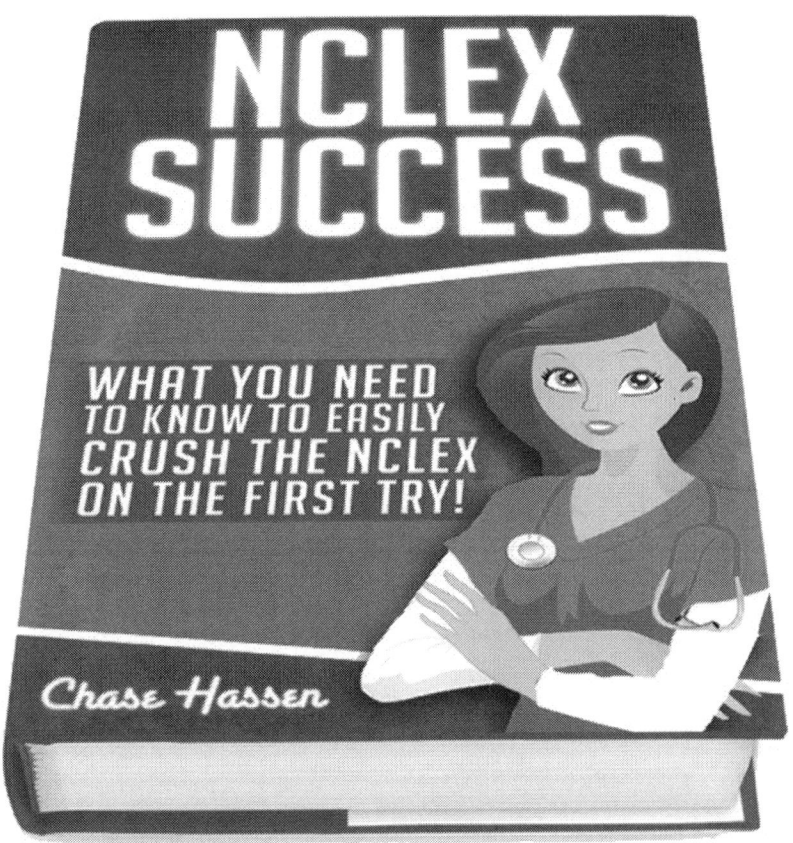

For a limited time, you can download this book for FREE.

Go To:

www.nursesuperhero.com/dc2

Table of Contents

Introduction 1

Unit 1: Essential Skills 5
    Chapter 1 The Metric System 7
    Chapter 2 Apothecary/Avoirdupois/Household Systems 9
    Chapter 3 Ratios 10
    Tool Shed (Conversion Factors) 11
    Chapter 4 Dimensional Analysis and Ratio Proportion 13
    Chapter 5 Rounding Numbers 17
    Chapter 6 Military Time (24-Hour Clock) 19

Unit 2: Auxiliary Subjects 21
    Chapter 7 Roman Numerals 23
    Chapter 8 Scientific Notation 29

Unit 3: Unit Conversions 32
    Chapter 9 Unit Conversions-The Basics 33
    Chapter 10 Unit Conversions Within the Metric System 35
    Chapter 11 Unit Conversions Within the Household System 37
    Chapter 12 Unit Conversions Between Metric, Household and Apothecary Systems 39
    Chapter 13 Unit Conversions Involving Pounds and Ounces 41
    Chapter 14 Unit Conversions Involving Hours and Minutes 43

Unit 4: Dosage Calculations 45
    Chapter 15 Dosage Calculations-The Basics 47
    Chapter 16 Dosage Calculations Level 1 53
    Chapter 17 Dosage Calculations Level 2 55
    Chapter 18 Dosage Calculations Level 3 59
    Chapter 19 Body Surface Area Dosing Calculations 63
    Chapter 20 Pediatric Dosage Calculations 67
    Chapter 21 Pediatric Maintenance Fluid Replacement Calculations 73

Unit 5: IV Flow Rate Calculations 75
    Chapter 22 IV Flow Rate Calculations-The Basics 77
    Chapter 23 IV Flow Rate Calculations Level 1 81
    Chapter 24 IV Flow Rate Calculations Level 2 83

Chapter 25 IV Flow Rate Adjustments 87

Chapter 26 Heparin Infusion and Adjustment Calculations 91

Unit 6: Percent and Ratio Strength Calculations 101

Chapter 27 Percent 103

Chapter 28 Percent Strength 105

Chapter 29 Percent Change 109

Chapter 30 Ratio Strength 113

Unit 7: Miscellaneous Subjects 115

Chapter 31 Reconstitution Calculations 117

Chapter 32 Concentrations and Dilutions... 121

Chapter 33 Milliequivalent Calculations 129

Chapter 34 Dosage Calculation Puzzles 133

Chapter 35 Self-Assessment Exam 135

A Final Note 143

List of Abbreviations and Symbols 144

Answers to Exercises 145

Chapter 5 Rounding Exercise 145

Chapter 6 Military Time Exercise.. 146

Chapter 7 Roman Numeral Exercise 147

Chapter 8 Scientific Notation Exercise.. 149

Chapter 10 Metric Conversion Exercise Using DA 151

Metric Conversion Exercise Using RP 152

Chapter 11 Household Conversion Exercise Using DA 153

Household Conversion Exercise Using RP.. 154

Chapter 12 Metric, Household and Apothecary Conversion Exercise Using DA................................ 155

Metric, Household and Apothecary Conversion Exercise Using RP 156

Chapter 13 Pounds and Ounces Conversion Exercise 157

Chapter 14 Hours and Minutes Conversion Exercise 158

Chapter 16 Dosage Calculations Level 1 Exercise.. 159

Chapter 17 Dosage Calculations Level 2 Exercise.. 160

Chapter 18 Dosage Calculations Level 3 Exercise.. 162

Chapter 19 BSA Calculation Exercise 164

Chapter 20 Pediatric Dosage Calculations Exercise ... 167
Chapter 21 Pediatric Maintenance Fluid Replacement Calculations ... 170
Chapter 23 IV Flow Rate Calculations Level 1 Exercise ... 172
Chapter 24 IV Flow Rate Calculations Level 2 Exercise ... 174
Chapter 25 IV Flow Rate Adjustments Exercise ... 177
Chapter 26 Heparin Infusion and Adjustment Calculations Exercise ... 180
Chapter 27 Percent Exercise ... 189
Chapter 28 Percent Strength Exercise ... 190
Chapter 29 Percent Change Exercise ... 192
Chapter 30 Ratio Strength Exercise ... 194
Chapter 31 Reconstitution Calculations Exercise ... 195
Chapter 32 Concentrations and Dilutions Exercise ... 197
Chapter 33 Milliequivalent Calculations Exercise ... 200
Chapter 34 Dosage Calculation Puzzles ... 202
Chapter 35 Self-Assessment Exam ... 205

Introduction

Welcome to the second edition of Dosage Calculations for Nursing Students. The second edition has all the basic information contained in the first edition along with many new chapters covering specific types of calculations. And yes, the second edition contains a few formulas which are necessary for some of the specialty calculations.

You are having some friends over for a BBQ and you will be grilling 24 hamburgers. You have plenty of hamburger patties, but you need 24 buns. You drive to the store and see that they are packaged 8 buns per package, so you pick up 3 packages. After getting home, you need to practice your dosage calculations and have the following problem. A provider has ordered 24 mg of a drug and you have on hand 8 mg/mL. How many mL will you administer? Did you need a hamburger bun formula to figure out how many packages of buns to buy? No, of course not, so why would you need a formula to calculate the dosage problem?

There are two main approaches to solving dosage calculations. You can either learn a long list of formulas, plug in the information from the problem and calculate the answer, or you can learn a few simple concepts and set up and solve the problem without resorting to formulas. This book takes the approach that it is safer and easier to learn what is happening in the problem and set up and solve it on your own.

Learning Objectives:

- The basics of the metric, apothecary, avoirdupois and household measurement systems.
- The three basic parts of dosage calculation problems.
- Setting up and solving dosage calculation problems using dimensional analysis and ratio proportion.
- Setting up and solving IV flow rate problems using dimensional analysis.
- Body surface area calculations.
- Dealing with percent, percent strength, percent change.
- Develop critical thinking skills required for specialty calculations.

What you will not learn:

- A long list of formulas.
- Moving the decimal point to the left or right.
- Multiplying or dividing by 1000, 30, 2.2 to convert units.
- Mathematically incorrect methods.

The book is divided into the following seven units:

Unit 1: Essential Skills:

You can't learn to drive a car if you don't understand the function of the steering wheel. The same applies to the following subjects when learning dosage calculations.

- The Metric System
- Apothecary/Avoirdupois/Household Systems
- Ratios
- Dimensional Analysis (DA) and Ratio Proportion (RP)
- Rounding Numbers
- Military Time

Unit 2: Auxiliary Subjects:

Unit 2 is short and covers Roman numerals and scientific notation, a couple of subjects which are probably not essential, but still somewhat important.

Unit 3: Unit Conversions

Unit 3 covers converting between and within the various systems of measurement using dimensional analysis and ratio proportion. The knowledge gained using DA and RP on these easy calculations will provide a firm foundation when moving on to dosage and IV flow rate calculations.

Unit 4: Dosage Calculations

Unit 4 builds on the knowledge gained in the previous units and covers dosage calculations, starting with the terminology and set up of problems, then progressing from easy, one-step, problems through multi-step problems. This unit also covers the specific topics of body surface area and pediatric dosage calculations.

Unit 5: IV Flow Rate Calculations

Unit 5 starts with the basic terminology and set up of IV flow rate problems, then moves on to simple and advanced problems. The topics of IV flow rate adjustments and heparin infusion calculations are also covered.

Unit 6: Percent and Ratio Strength Calculations

Percent, percent strength, percent change and ratio strength are important topics covered in Unit 6. These topics are not difficult if a few basic concepts are understood.

Unit 7: Miscellaneous Subjects

The following subjects are covered in unit 7:

- Reconstitution Calculations
- Concentrations and Dilutions
- Milliequivalent Calculations
- Dosage Calculations Puzzles
- Self-Assessment Exam

General Terminology Used in this Book:

- **Number: Includes integers, decimal numbers, and fractions.**
    - Integer: All positive and negative whole numbers and zero.
        - Examples: -4, -3, 0, 2, 25
    - Decimal Number: A number which includes a decimal point.
        - Examples: 25.3, 0.05
    - Fraction: A number represented as a/b where a and b are both integers, with the exception that b cannot be 0.
        - Examples: 1/2, 3/4, 7/8, -1/2
- **Unit: Unit of measurement.**
    - Examples: mg, mL, kg, L.

A Few Important Notes:

- Always include all units of measurement (mg, g, L, mL, etc.) in the calculations.
    - The units are the most important part of the calculation. The numbers only go along for the ride.
- Set the calculations up mathematically correct.
    - 0.25 X 100% = 25% **not** 0.25 X 100 = 25%
- Use a space between the number and the unit.
    - 5 mL not 5mL
- Always use leading zeros on decimal numbers which are less than 1.
    - 0.5 mg not .5 mg. It is easy to misread .5 mg as 5 mg.
- Always avoid trailing zeros after whole numbers.
    - 5 mg not 5.0 mg. It is easy to misread 5.0 mg as 50 mg.
- Single quantities in equations can be expressed by themselves or as a ratio with 1 in the denominator. $2 \text{ h} \left(\frac{60 \text{ min}}{\text{h}}\right) = 120 \text{ min}$ can be written $\frac{2 \text{ h}}{1} \left(\frac{60 \text{ min}}{\text{h}}\right) = 120 \text{ min}$.
- Use mcg for microgram, not µg, as µg can be mistaken for mg.

Rounding rules for this book, unless otherwise stated:

- In general, round calculations at the end.
- All drops/minute calculations are to be rounded to the nearest full drop.
- All mL/h calculations are to be rounded to the nearest tenth mL/h unless otherwise stated.
- mL doses less than 1 mL are rounded to the nearest hundredth mL.
- mL doses greater than or equal to 1 mL are rounded to the nearest tenth mL.
- When rounding the final answer to the nearest tenth or hundredth, if the final digit after the decimal point is zero, omit it. This is done to avoid trailing zeros.

Enjoy the book!

-Brad Wojcik & Chase Hassen

Unit 1: Essential Skills

As with any subject, certain basic skills are required before delving into the actual subject matter. The following subjects are covered in Unit 1.

Chapter 1: The Metric System
Summary: An overview of the metric system as it relates to nursing.
Importance: 10/10.

Chapter 2: Apothecary/Avoirdupois/Household Systems
Summary: An overview of other systems of measurement encountered in nursing.
Importance: 10/10

Chapter 3: Ratios
Summary: An explanation of ratios and their role in dosage calculations. Virtually every dosage calculation, IV flow rate calculation and unit conversion will involve use of one or more ratios, and it is vitally important that you fully understand them.
Importance: 10/10

Chapter 4: Dimensional Analysis and Ratio Proportion
Summary: A basic explanation of dimensional analysis and ratio proportion. It is important to understand the math behind dosage calculations and why these methods work.
Importance: 10/10

Chapter 5: Rounding Numbers
Summary: An explanation of rounding numbers. As most dosage calculations involve rounding, a thorough understanding of this subject is vital.
Importance: 10/10

Chapter 6: Military Time
Summary: An explanation of military time (24-hour clock).
Importance: 10/10

Chapter 1
The Metric System

- The metric system is the predominant system of measurement used in nursing.
- The primary base units used in nursing are gram, liter, and meter.
- Each of the base units can be multiplied or divided by powers of 10 to form larger or smaller units.
- Prefixes are placed before the base units to denote the larger and smaller units.
- The first table below lists the most important metric units used in nursing.

The Metric System Basics for Nurses

Prefix	Symbol	Multiple of base	Weight	Volume	Length
micro	mc	1/1,000,000	mcg		
milli	m	1/1000	mg	mL	mm
centi	c	1/100			cm
deci	d	1/10		dL	
		Base Unit	g (gram)	L (liter)	m (meter)
kilo	k	1000	kg		km

Approximate Equivalents to Selected Metric Units

Weight Unit	Approximate Equivalent	Volume Unit	Approximate Equivalent	Length Unit	Approximate Equivalent
mcg	1 ant leg?	mL	20 drops	mm	1/25 inch
mg	6 grains of salt	dL	3 1/3 fl oz	cm	4/10 inch
g	1 large paperclip	L	1 quart	m	1 yard
kg	2.2 lb			km	6/10 mile

Metric Prefixes Between 10^{18} and 10^{-18}

Prefix	Symbol	Multiplication Factor	Exponent
exa	E	1000000000000000000	10^{18}
peta	P	1000000000000000	10^{15}
tera	T	1000000000000	10^{12}
giga	G	1000000000	10^{9}
mega	M	1000000	10^{6}
kilo	k	1000	10^{3}
hecto	h	100	10^{2}
deca	da	10	10^{1}
	Base Unit	1	10^{0}
deci	d	0.1	10^{-1}
centi	c	0.01	10^{-2}
milli	m	0.001	10^{-3}
micro	mc	0.000001	10^{-6}
nano	n	0.000000001	10^{-9}
pico	p	0.000000000001	10^{-12}
femto	f	0.000000000000001	10^{-15}
atto	a	0.000000000000000001	10^{-18}

It is essential that you know the following equivalences. If you run into other units such as ng, you can always reference the above chart.

- 1 kg = 1000 g
- 1 g = 1000 mg
- 1 mg = 1000 mcg
- 1 L = 1000 mL
- 1 dL = 100 mL
- 1 m = 100 cm
- 1 cm = 10 mm

These equations, along with some others, will form the basis for the ratios which you will learn about in Chapter 3.

Chapter 2
Apothecary/Avoirdupois/Household Systems

- These systems are rarely used in nursing today, but there are a few units and key points which should be learned.
- Weight Units:
  - Grain (gr): Technically 64.8 mg, but NCLEX rounds to 60 mg.
  - Ounce (oz): Technically 28.3 g, but usually rounded to 30 g.
  - Pound (lb): Contains 16 oz. Usually rounded to 454 g.
- Volume Units:
  - Fluidram/fluid dram: Technically 3.7 mL, but usually rounded to 5 mL.
  - Fluid ounce (fl oz): Technically 29.6 mL, but usually rounded to 30 mL
  - Pint (pt): 16 fluid ounces. Technically 473 mL, but usually rounded to 480 mL.
    - ✓ 2 pints = 1 quart
    - ✓ 4 quarts = 1 gallon
  - Teaspoonful (tsp): 5 mL (Note: Should be measured with a measuring device, not kitchen silverware.)
  - Tablespoonful (tbs): 15 mL (See note for teaspoonful.)
  - Cup: 8 fl oz which is usually rounded to 240 mL

Important Units with Rounded Metric Equivalents

Apothecary Volume	Household Volume	Metric Volume
1 fluidram /fluid dram	1 teaspoonful (tsp)	5 mL
1 fluid ounce	2 tablespoonfuls (tbs)	30 mL
8 fluid ounces	1 cup	240 mL
16 fluid ounces	1 pint (pt)	480 mL (473 mL)
	1 tablespoonful	15 mL
Apothecary Weight		**Metric Weight**
1 grain (gr)		60 mg
Avoirdupois Weight	**Household Weight**	**Metric Weight**
1 ounce (oz)	1 ounce (oz)	30 g
1 pound (lb)	1 pound (lb)	454 g (0.454 kg)

It is important that you know the following equivalences.

1 tsp = 5 mL	1 cup = 240 mL	1 lb = 16 oz
1 tbs = 15 mL	1 pt = 16 fl oz	1 lb = 454 g
1 fl oz = 30 mL	1 gr = 60 mg	1 oz = 30 g
1 cup = 8 fl oz	1 kg = 2.2 lb	

Dosage Calculations for Nursing Students-Second Edition

Chapter 3
Ratios

If you Google "ratios" you will see a lot of different definitions. What we will be dealing with in this book is dimensioned ratios, that is ratios which have units of measurement attached.

In Chapters 1 and 2 you were asked to learn the following equivalences:

1 kg = 1000 g	1 tsp = 5 mL
1 g = 1000 mg	1 fl oz = 30 mL
1 mg = 1000 mcg	1 gr = 60 mg
1 L = 1000 mL	1 lb = 454 g
1 dL = 100 mL	1 kg = 2.2 lb
1 m = 100 cm	1 lb = 16 oz
1 cm = 10 mm	

Looking at 1 kg = 1000 g, we can say that there are 1000 g per 1 kg and write the following ratio:

$$\frac{1000 \text{ g}}{1 \text{ kg}}$$

We can also say that there is 1 kg per 1000 g and write the following ratio:

$$\frac{1 \text{ kg}}{1000 \text{ g}}$$

This is important! 5 = 5 and 1 kg = 1000 g. Anything, except zero, divided by itself, or something equal to itself equals 1. $\frac{5}{5} = 1, \frac{1 \text{ kg}}{1000 \text{ g}} = 1$

Why is it important to know that $\frac{1 \text{ kg}}{1000 \text{ g}} = 1$? Because we can multiply anything by 1, or a form of 1, and not change its value. If you are asked to calculate the number of kg in 5200 g, you can simply multiply 5200 g by $\frac{1 \text{ kg}}{1000 \text{ g}}$. The g's will cancel out giving you 5.2 kg. Think of the ratios as tools which are used to change the units of what you are given into the units of the answer. The following chart contains a list of ratios (conversion factors) you can use in your calculations.

Tool Shed (Conversion Factors)

These conversion factors equal 1 and can be flipped upside down, if needed.

Metric Weight: $\left(\frac{1 \text{ g}}{1000 \text{ mg}}\right) \left(\frac{1000 \text{ mg}}{1 \text{ g}}\right) \left(\frac{1 \text{ kg}}{1000 \text{ g}}\right) \left(\frac{1000 \text{ g}}{1 \text{ kg}}\right) \left(\frac{1 \text{ mg}}{1000 \text{ mcg}}\right) \left(\frac{1000 \text{ mcg}}{1 \text{ mg}}\right)$

Metric Volume: $\left(\frac{1 \text{ L}}{1000 \text{ mL}}\right) \left(\frac{1000 \text{ mL}}{1 \text{ L}}\right) \left(\frac{1 \text{ dL}}{100 \text{ mL}}\right) \left(\frac{100 \text{ mL}}{1 \text{ dL}}\right)$

Metric - U.S. Weight: $\left(\frac{30 \text{ g}}{1 \text{ oz}}\right) \left(\frac{1 \text{ oz}}{30 \text{ g}}\right) \left(\frac{2.2 \text{ lb}}{1 \text{ kg}}\right) \left(\frac{1 \text{ kg}}{2.2 \text{ lb}}\right) \left(\frac{1 \text{ lb}}{454 \text{ g}}\right) \left(\frac{454 \text{ g}}{1 \text{ lb}}\right)$

Metric – U.S. Volume: $\left(\frac{1 \text{ tsp}}{5 \text{ mL}}\right) \left(\frac{5 \text{ mL}}{1 \text{ tsp}}\right) \left(\frac{1 \text{ fl oz}}{30 \text{ mL}}\right) \left(\frac{30 \text{ mL}}{1 \text{ fl oz}}\right) \left(\frac{1 \text{ pt}}{480 \text{ mL}}\right) \left(\frac{480 \text{ mL}}{1 \text{ pt}}\right) \left(\frac{1 \text{ tbs}}{15 \text{ mL}}\right) \left(\frac{15 \text{ mL}}{1 \text{ tbs}}\right)$

U.S. Volume: $\left(\frac{1 \text{ tbs}}{3 \text{ tsp}}\right) \left(\frac{3 \text{ tsp}}{1 \text{ tbs}}\right) \left(\frac{16 \text{ fl oz}}{1 \text{ pt}}\right) \left(\frac{1 \text{ pt}}{16 \text{ fl oz}}\right) \left(\frac{1 \text{ qt}}{2 \text{ pt}}\right) \left(\frac{8 \text{ fl oz}}{1 \text{ cup}}\right) \left(\frac{1 \text{ cup}}{8 \text{ fl oz}}\right) \left(\frac{1 \text{ gal}}{4 \text{ qt}}\right) \left(\frac{4 \text{ qt}}{1 \text{ gal}}\right)$

Metric Length: $\left(\frac{1 \text{ m}}{100 \text{ cm}}\right) \left(\frac{100 \text{ cm}}{1 \text{ m}}\right) \left(\frac{1 \text{ cm}}{10 \text{ mm}}\right) \left(\frac{10 \text{ mm}}{1 \text{ cm}}\right)$

Metric - U.S. Length: $\left(\frac{1 \text{ in}}{2.54 \text{ cm}}\right) \left(\frac{2.54 \text{ cm}}{1 \text{ in}}\right)$

Apothecary - Metric Volume: $\left(\frac{1 \text{ fl dram}}{5 \text{ mL}}\right) \left(\frac{5 \text{ mL}}{1 \text{ fl dram}}\right) \left(\frac{1 \text{ fl oz}}{30 \text{ mL}}\right) \left(\frac{30 \text{ mL}}{1 \text{ fl oz}}\right)$

Apothecary - Metric Weight: $\left(\frac{60 \text{ mg}}{1 \text{ gr}}\right) \left(\frac{1 \text{ gr}}{60 \text{ mg}}\right)$

Percent: $\left(\frac{1}{100\%}\right) \left(\frac{100\%}{1}\right) (100\%)$

Time: $\left(\frac{60 \text{ sec}}{1 \text{ min}}\right) \left(\frac{1 \text{ min}}{60 \text{ sec}}\right) \left(\frac{60 \text{ min}}{1 \text{ h}}\right) \left(\frac{1 \text{ h}}{60 \text{ min}}\right) \left(\frac{24 \text{ h}}{1 \text{ d}}\right) \left(\frac{1 \text{ d}}{24 \text{ h}}\right)$

Temperature: °F = (1.8 °C) + 32°

What about all the other ratios you encounter in dosage calculations? How about amoxicillin 250 mg/5 mL? Does 250 mg = 5 mL and $\frac{250 \text{ mg}}{5 \text{ mL}} = 1$? Yes, if a ratio is given to you in a problem, it will equal 1. The patient will receive the same amount of amoxicillin weather 250 mg or 5 mL of the suspension is administered.

Summary

- All the conversion factors listed in the Tool Shed always hold true and can be used whenever needed. All conversion factors can be flipped upside down if need and they always equal 1.
- All ratios given in a dosage problem equal 1 and can be flipped upside down if needed. Examples include drug strengths (100 mg/1 mL, 500 mg/ 1 tablet), drop factors (15 drops/ 1 mL), and weight-based dosages (10 mg/kg).

Chapter 4, Dimensional Analysis and Ratio Proportion will go into detail on how to put your knowledge of ratios to work solving problems. Understanding the information in this unit is half the battle. The rest is easy.

Before proceeding to Chapter 4, please read and initial the following:

I understand:

- All conversion factors (1000 mg/g, 60 min/h, 2.2 lb/kg, etc.) equal 1 and can be flipped upside down if needed.
- All ratios given in dosage problems (100 mg/mL, 250 mg/tab, 100 mL/h, etc.) equal 1 and can be flipped upside down if needed.

Initial_____ **Date**_____

Ok, that was a little extreme, but now you won't forget.

Chapter 4
Dimensional Analysis and Ratio Proportion

If you know the basics of the metric, apothecary, avoirdupois and household systems of measurements and you know that all the ratios you will be working with equal 1 and can be flipped upside down when needed, then you are ready to learn the most important chapter in the book.

Terminology:

- **Dimensional Analysis (DA):** A powerful method of solving problems in nursing, pharmacy, chemistry, physics, and engineering in which a given is multiplied by one or more ratios, which equal 1, to change the units of the given into the units of the answer.
- **Ratio Proportion (RP):** A method widely used by the medical community to solve problems by comparing two ratios.

It is extremely important to fully understand everything in this chapter.

Most of the calculations encountered in nursing involve nothing more than changing the units from what is given to the units desired. These include:

- Unit Conversions
- Dosage Calculations
- IV Flow Rate Calculations
- Percent, Percent Strength, and Ratio Strength Calculations
- Milliequivalent Calculations

These calculations can all be solved using DA or RP.

Think of these not as five different types of calculations, but as a single type of calculation involving five different types of units.

These problems all have the same three parts:

- **The Units of the Answer:** Think of it as the destination.
- **A Given:** This is what is given to start the problem and what is changed into the answer.
- **One or More Ratios:** These are the tools used to change the units of the given into the units of the answer.

Example 1 using DA: Convert 4.5 g to mg.

- The units of the answer are mg. This is the destination.
- The given is 4.5 g. This is the starting point.
- The ratio is 1000 mg/g. This is the tool to change g to mg.

- Start by listing the starting point and destination. This will help when placing the ratio(s).

4.5 g = mg

- Place the ratio with the units of the answer on top and the units to be canceled on the bottom. Multiply the given by the ratio. The grams cancel out, leaving mg in the answer.

$$4.5\ \mathbf{g}\left(\frac{\mathbf{1000\ mg}}{\mathbf{g}}\right) = \mathbf{4500\ mg\ or}\ \frac{\mathbf{4.5\ g}}{\mathbf{1}}\left(\frac{\mathbf{1000\ mg}}{\mathbf{g}}\right) = \mathbf{4500\ mg}$$

Example 2 using DA: A patient is prescribed 400 mg. The drug is available in a strength of 200 mg/mL. How many mL will be ad

A patient is perscribed 400 mg.
The drug is available in a
Strength of 200 mg/mL
How many mL will be administered?

400mg = mL

$400\,mg\left(\frac{1\,mL}{200\,mg}\right) = 2\,mL$

- The units of the answer are mL
- The given is 400 mg.
- The ratio is 200 mg/mL.
- Start by listing the starting poi

4

- Place the ratio with the units ... canceled on the bottom. Multiply the given by ... g mL.

- In this case, the ratio was flipp ... on the bottom.

Key Points about the Ratios

- **The ratios always equal 1**. Since 1000 mg = 1 g, $\frac{1000\ \text{mg}}{1\ \text{g}} = 1$ (In this book, this type of ratio is called an "off the shelf" ratio because it is always true. There are always 1000 mg in a g.)

  In example 2, it is stated the drug's strength is 200 mg/mL. For this problem, it can be stated that 1 mL = 200 mg. $\frac{1\ \text{mL}}{200\ \text{mg}} = 1$ and $\frac{200\ \text{mg}}{1\ \text{mL}} = 1$. (In this book, this type of ratio is called a "custom ratio" because it only holds true for the problem at hand. There are not always 200 mg/mL, only if the problem states it.)
- **The ratios can be flipped upside down if needed.** $\frac{\mathbf{1000\ mg}}{\mathbf{1\ g}} = \frac{\mathbf{1\ g}}{\mathbf{1000\ mg}} = \mathbf{1}$

The above two examples were solved using the dimensional analysis method. An explanation of the ratio proportion method follows.

The Ratio Proportion Method

The ratio proportion method is the other method used to solve the problems in this unit. Using the ratio proportion method, also called the ratio and proportion method, two ratios are set up that are proportional (equal) to each other and the unknown is solved for. Using the above examples:

Example 1 using RP: Convert 4.5 g into mg.

- The RP method uses two ratios: one ratio containing the unknown and the given, the other ratio serving as a reference ratio.

$$\frac{x \text{ mg}}{4.5 \text{ g}} = \frac{1000 \text{ mg}}{1 \text{ g}}$$

- The easiest way to solve for x mg is to cross multiply (4.5 g) (1000 mg) then divide by 1 g, resulting in the answer of **4500 mg**.

Example 2 using RP: A patient is prescribed 400 mg. The drug is available in a strength of 200 mg/mL. How many mL will be administered?

$$\frac{x \text{ mL}}{400 \text{ mg}} = \frac{1 \text{ mL}}{200 \text{ mg}}$$

- Solving for x mL: (400 mg) (1 mL)/200 mg = 2 mL

When using the ratio proportion method, both numerators must have the same units and both denominators must have the same units.

For simple one step problems, there is not a lot of difference between DA and RP as far as ease of use or safety. Now consider the following problem, which involves two ratios, solved using both DA and RP.

Example 3 using DA: A patient has been prescribed 150 mg of a drug which is available in 10 mL vials containing 2.5 g of drug. How many mL should be administered?

- The units of the answer are mL.
- The given is 150 mg.
- The ratios are 2.5 g/10 mL and 1000 mg/g.

$$150 \text{ mg} \left(\frac{1 \text{ g}}{1000 \text{ mg}}\right)\left(\frac{10 \text{ mL}}{2.5 \text{ g}}\right) = 0.6 \text{ mL}$$

Dosage Calculations for Nursing Students-Second Edition

Example 3 using RP: A patient has been prescribed 150 mg of a drug which is available in 10 mL vials containing 2.5 g of drug. How many mL should be administered?

- Step 1) Convert 150 mg to g.

$$\frac{x\,g}{150\,mg} = \frac{1\,g}{1000\,mg}$$

  ➢ Solving for x g yields 0.15 g.

- Step 2) Calculate the dose in mL needed to supply 0.15 g.

$$\frac{x\,mL}{0.15\,g} = \frac{10\,mL}{2.5\,g}$$

  ➢ Solving for x mL yields 0.6 mL

As you can see, each step requires an additional calculation starting with the answer from the previous calculation.

It is the authors' belief that the dimensional analysis method is superior to the ratio proportion method for problems involving more than one step.

- Using dimensional analysis, the problem can be set up in one step and checked for accuracy by canceling out the units before any calculations are performed.
- Using the ratio proportion method, several problems may have to be set up, complicating the problem and introducing sources of error.
- A small pile of gravel can be moved with an "RP shovel" but climb into a "DA bulldozer" to move a large pile.

Going forward, both the DA and RP method will be shown for the simple unit conversion problems and simple dosage calculation problems, but only DA will be shown for the other problems.

---

150 mg to g.

So we know 1g = 60mg.
therefore 150 ÷ 60 = 2.5g.

If 10ml is in vials of 2.5g
then 10ml should be given

1g = 1000mg.

2.5g = 2500 mg.

150mg - 1.5g /

10mL - 2.5g

150 ÷ 1000 = 0.15

0.15g ÷ 2.5 = 0.6ml.

The Ratio Proportion Method

The ratio proportion method is the other method used to solve the problems in this unit. Using the ratio proportion method, also called the ratio and proportion method, two ratios are set up that are proportional (equal) to each other and the unknown is solved for. Using the above examples:

Example 1 using RP: Convert 4.5 g into mg.

- The RP method uses two ratios: one ratio containing the unknown and the given, the other ratio serving as a reference ratio.

$$\frac{x \text{ mg}}{4.5 \text{ g}} = \frac{1000 \text{ mg}}{1 \text{ g}}$$

- The easiest way to solve for x mg is to cross multiply (4.5 g) (1000 mg) then divide by 1 g, resulting in the answer of **4500 mg**.

Example 2 using RP: A patient is prescribed 400 mg. The drug is available in a strength of 200 mg/mL. How many mL will be administered?

$$\frac{x \text{ mL}}{400 \text{ mg}} = \frac{1 \text{ mL}}{200 \text{ mg}}$$

- Solving for x mL: (400 mg) (1 mL)/200 mg = 2 mL

When using the ratio proportion method, both numerators must have the same units and both denominators must have the same units.

For simple one step problems, there is not a lot of difference between DA and RP as far as ease of use or safety. Now consider the following problem, which involves two ratios, solved using both DA and RP.

Example 3 using DA: A patient has been prescribed 150 mg of a drug which is available in 10 mL vials containing 2.5 g of drug. How many mL should be administered?

- The units of the answer are mL.
- The given is 150 mg.
- The ratios are 2.5 g/10 mL and 1000 mg/g.

$$150 \text{ mg} \left(\frac{1 \text{ g}}{1000 \text{ mg}}\right)\left(\frac{10 \text{ mL}}{2.5 \text{ g}}\right) = 0.6 \text{ mL}$$

Example 3 using RP: A patient has been prescribed 150 mg of a drug which is available in 10 mL vials containing 2.5 g of drug. How many mL should be administered?

- Step 1) Convert 150 mg to g.

$$\frac{x\,g}{150\,mg} = \frac{1\,g}{1000\,mg}$$

  ➤ Solving for x g yields 0.15 g.
- Step 2) Calculate the dose in mL needed to supply 0.15 g.

$$\frac{x\,mL}{0.15\,g} = \frac{10\,mL}{2.5\,g}$$

  ➤ Solving for x mL yields 0.6 mL

As you can see, each step requires an additional calculation starting with the answer from the previous calculation.

It is the authors' belief that the dimensional analysis method is superior to the ratio proportion method for problems involving more than one step.

- Using dimensional analysis, the problem can be set up in one step and checked for accuracy by canceling out the units before any calculations are performed.
- Using the ratio proportion method, several problems may have to be set up, complicating the problem and introducing sources of error.
- A small pile of gravel can be moved with an "RP shovel" but climb into a "DA bulldozer" to move a large pile.

Going forward, both the DA and RP method will be shown for the simple unit conversion problems and simple dosage calculation problems, but only DA will be shown for the other problems.

Chapter 5
Rounding Numbers

Many times, calculated answers will have more decimal places than needed or desired and rounding will be required. To round a number:

- Identify the digit occupying the place to be rounded to. For example, if asked to round to the nearest tenth, you would look at the 8 in the following example.

3	5	6	.	8	1	9
Hundreds	Tens	Ones	Decimal Point	Tenths	Hundredths	Thousandths

- Look at the digit following the digit being rounded. In the above example, this is the 1.
- If the following digit is 0,1,2,3, or 4, all digits following the digit being rounded are dropped and you are finished. In the above example, the 1 and 9 are dropped, leaving 356.8 as the rounded number.
- If the following digit is 5,6,7,8, or 9, all digits following the digit being rounded are dropped, and the digit is increase by 1. In rounding the number 149.379 to the nearest tenth, the 7 and 9 are dropped and the 3 is increased to 4, leaving 149.4 as the rounded number.

IMPORTANT: When rounding numbers, look ONLY at the first digit after the digit being rounded. All other digits are irrelevant.

Example: Round to the nearest tenth.

- 6.759 rounded is 6.8 (Look only at the 5; the 9 is irrelevant.)
- 10.248 rounded is 10.2 (Look only at the 4; the 8 is irrelevant.)
- 0.38999 rounded is 0.4 (Look only at the 8; the 9's are irrelevant.)

Example: Round to the nearest hundredth.

- 89.523 rounded is 89.52
- 0.59788 rounded is 0.60
- 7.2395 rounded is 7.24

10th, 1st after decimal   **Rounding Exercise**   100th, 2nd after dec.

Problem	Round to the Nearest Tenth	Rounded Number	Problem	Round to the Nearest Hundredth	Rounded Number
Example	3.054	3.1	Example	78.386	78.39
1	121.16	121.2 ✓	26	8.875	8.88 ✓
2	4.37	4.4 ✓	27	3.295	3.30 ✓
3	10.26	10.3 ✓	28	5.111	5.11 ✓
4	89.43	89.4 ✓	28	35.589	35.59 ✓
5	6.57	6.6 ✓	30	9.598	9.60 ✓
6	87.449	87.4 ✓	31	0.297	0.30 ✓
7	0.3256	0.3 ✓	32	6.205	6.21 ✓
8	2.98	3.0 ✓	33	6.393	6.40 ✓
9	708.32	708.3 ✓	34	58.451	58.46 ✓
10	29.99	30.0 ✓	35	2.782	2.79 ✓
11	5.06	5.1 ✓	36	5.433	5.43 ✓
12	23.598	23.6 ✓	37	4.554	4.56 ✓
13	78.53	78.5 ✓	38	2.256	2.26 ✓
14	5.44	5.4 ✓	39	1.874	1.88 ✓
15	78.3	78.3 ✓	40	3.987	3.99 ✓
16	10.01	10.0 ✓	41	9.672	9.68 ✓
17	53.247	53.2 ✓	42	3.3595	3.36 ✓
18	0.88	0.9 ✓	43	1.005	1.01 ✓
19	2.22	2.2 ✓	44	4.956	4.96 ✓
20	9.355	9.3 ✗ 9.4	45	1.8954	1.90 ✓
21	9.11	9.1 ✓	46	89.548	89.55 ✓
22	9.78	9.8 ✓	47	0.987	0.99 ✓
23	78.59	78.6 ✓	48	6.523	6.52 ✓
24	76.203	76.2 ✓	49	2.212	2.21 ✓
25	22.56	22.6 ✓	50	4.228	4.23 ✓

Dosage Calculations for Nursing Students-Second Edition

Chapter 6
Military Time (24-Hour Clock)

Hospitals typically use military time rather than civilian time (12 hour-AM/PM).

- Military time is based on a 24-hour clock.
- The following chart gives the corresponding military times and civilian times.

Civilian Time	Military Time (24-Hour)	Civilian Time	Military Time (24-Hour)
Midnight	0000 or 2400	Noon	1200
12:01 AM	0001	12:01 PM	1201
1:00 AM	0100	1:00 PM	1300
2:00 AM	0200	2:00 PM	1400
3:00 AM	0300	3:00 PM	1500
4:00 AM	0400	4:00 PM	1600
5:00 AM	0500	5:00 PM	1700
6:00 AM	0600	6:00 PM	1800
7:00 AM	0700	7:00 PM	1900
8:00 AM	0800	8:00 PM	2000
9:00 AM	0900	9:00 PM	2100
10:00 AM	1000	10:00 PM	2200
11:00 AM	1100	11:00 PM	2300

- The times between 1:00 AM and 12:59 PM are the same in military time as they are in civilian time. Just remove the colon and add a zero in front of the numbers below 10.
- For times between 1:00 PM and 11:59 PM, add 12 hours to convert to military time.
- For times between 12:00 Midnight and 12:59 AM, subtract 12 hours.

Military Time Exercise

Convert the following civilian times to military time.

1) 3:15 AM   03.15 ✓

2) 9:25 PM   21.25 ✓

3) 8:13 AM   08.13 ✓

4) 10:23 PM   22.23 ✓

5) 4:49 AM   04.49 ✓

Convert the following military times to civilian times.

6) 0422   4:22 AM ✓

7) 2215   10:15 PM ✓

8) 0905   9:05 AM ✓

9) 0710   7:10 AM ✓

10) 1310   01:10 PM ✓

11) You started work at 0700 and you ended work at 1630. You didn't get any lunch or breaks (poor you). How many hours did you work? 9h 30m ✓

12) An IV was started at 1100 and ended at 3:30 PM. How many hours did it run?
4h 30m ✓

13) You have the weekend off. You started watching your favorite Netflix series at 0830 on Saturday morning and finished at 0030 on Sunday. How many hours did you sit on the couch watching TV? 12h ✗ 16h

14) A patient is admitted at 0600 Monday morning and is discharged at 0800 the following morning. How many hours did the patient spend in the hospital?
26h ✓

Dosage Calculations for Nursing Students-Second Edition

Unit 2: Auxiliary Subjects

Unit 2 contains a couple of subjects which didn't make it into the essential skills unit but may come up occasionally in dosage calculations. You should know the basics of Roman numerals and scientific notation, if not for nursing, for everyday life.

Chapter 7: Roman Numerals
Summary: An explanation of the Roman numeral system.
Importance: 5/10. You should, at the very least, know Roman numerals for numbers 1-30.

Chapter 8: Scientific Notation
Summary: An explanation of scientific notation, which is an easier method of writing very large and very small numbers.
Importance: 5/10. You can probably skip this chapter and use it as a reference if needed.

Roman Numeral

SS ½
I 1
V 5
X 10
L 50
C 100
D 500
M 1000

* If smaller numeral is placed before a larger numeral, the smaller numeral is subtracted from the larger.

i.e IV = 4

the I is subtracted from V (5-1).

Only I, X and C may be subtracted from a larger numeral.
The "five" numerals (V, L, D) may not be subtracted from larger numeral.

45 is written XLV

Chapter 7
Roman Numerals

- The decimal number system, also called the Arabic number system, is a positional number system in which the position of the digit determines its value. The 2 in 521 represents 20, but the 2 in 245 represents 200.
- The Roman numeral system is an additive and subtractive system in which the value of a numeral remains constant. The C in CXX represents a value of 100, just as the C in CLXV represents 100.

Roman Numerals and Their Values

Roman Numeral	Value	Memory Hints
SS	1/2	Short stack of pancakes, which is about half a regular stack.
I	1	Easy to remember because it looks like a 1.
V	5	Your hand with your fingers together and thumb apart forms a V.
X	10	Think of it as two V's, one on top of the other.
L	50	Think of **L**asso. It has 5 letters and ends in O (50).
C	100	Think of **C**entury or **C**-note.
D	500	Imagine 500 **D**ogs in your house, all barking and running around.
M	1000	Think of **M**illennium.

Rules for Forming Roman Numerals

1) Start from the left with the largest numeral and work down to the smallest on the right.

2) No more than three of the same numeral in a row. 40 cannot be written XXXX.

3) If a smaller numeral is placed before a larger numeral, the smaller numeral is subtracted from the larger numeral. For example, IV is 4; the I is subtracted from V (5-1).

4) Only I, X, and C may be subtracted from a larger numeral. The "five" numerals (V, L, D) may not be subtracted from a larger numeral. 45 is written XLV, not VL.

5) When a smaller numeral is subtracted from a larger numeral, the smaller numeral can be no less than one tenth of the larger numeral. IX is 9, but IL is not permitted for 49, nor IC for 99. 49 is written XLIX and 99 is written XCIX. Only one numeral at a time may be subtracted and only from one other numeral. IIX is not permitted for 8, nor IXX for 19.

6) Always use the largest numerals possible. 15 is written XV, not VVV, even though writing three V's does not break rule #2.

These rules may seem complicated, but with a little practice Roman numerals are easy if you learn the following tips.

- A smaller numeral must be subtracted from a larger numeral only if the number contains a 4 or 9. 246 is written CCXLVI with the X being subtracted from the L. 2386 is written MMCCCLXXXVI, with no subtraction involved.
- When one numeral is subtracted from another, think of them as a unit. Think of IV as 4, not 5-1, XL as 40, not 50-10, etc.
- Learn the following table to be able to quickly form any Roman numeral.

1000	M	100	C	10	X	1	I
2000	MM	200	CC	20	XX	2	II
3000	MMM	300	CCC	30	XXX	3	III
		400	CD	40	XL	4	IV
		500	D	50	L	5	V
		600	DC	60	LX	6	VI
		700	DCC	70	LXX	7	VII
		800	DCCC	80	LXXX	8	VIII
		900	CM	90	XC	9	IX
						1/2	SS

Example: Convert 2648 to a Roman numeral.

- Separate out the 1000's, 100's, 10's, and 1's and place the corresponding Roman numeral next to them.

2000	MM
600	DC
40	XL
8	VIII

- Line up the Roman numerals in order starting with the largest.
  ➢ MMDCXLVIII

Example: Convert MCMXXXIV to a number.

- Separate out the 1000's, 100's, 10's, and 1's and place the corresponding number next to them.

M	1000
CM	900
XXX	30
IV	4

- Total the numbers.
  ➢ 1934

Roman Numeral Exercise

1) You must know the eight basic Roman numerals and their number counterparts: SS, I, V, X, L, C, D, M. Fill in the blanks in the following table.

Roman Numeral	Number	Number	Roman Numeral
SS	½ 0.5	1/2 (0.5)	SS
I	1	1	I
V	5	5	V
X	10	10	X
L	50	50	L
C	100	100	C
D	500	500	D
M	1000	1000	M

2) Fill in the blanks with the corresponding Roman numerals or numbers.

50	L	C	100
100	C	5	V
1/2	SS	10	X
X	10	L	50
M	1000	I	1
5	V	X	10
V	5	D	500
500	D	M	1000
L	50	X	10
SS	1/2	V	5
1000	M	L	50
1	I	C	100
D	500	5	V
L	50	50	L
M	1000	1000	M
10	X	100	C

3) Fill in the blanks with the corresponding Roman numerals.

1000	M	100	C	10	X	1	I
2000	MM	200	CC	20	XX	2	II
3000	MMM	300	CCC	30	XXX	3	III
		400	CD	40	XL	4	IV
		500	D	50	L	5	V
		600	DC	60	LX	6	VI
		700	DCC	70	LXX	7	VII
		800	DCCC	80	LXXX	8	VIII
		900	CM	90	XC	9	IX
						1/2	SS

4) Fill in the blanks with the corresponding number or Roman numeral.

10		LXX	
30		20	
400		CCC	
DC		CD	
2000		CM	
8		700	
XC		50	
40		20	
60		LXXX	
200		DCC	
900		600	
IV		CC	
III		9	
SS		4	

Write the corresponding Roman numerals or numbers:

Example: Write 2462 as a Roman numeral.

2000	MM
400	CD
60	LX
2	II

- Line up the Roman numerals in order starting with the largest.
  - MMCDLXII

Example: Write MDCLXVII as a number.

M	1000
DC	600
LX	60
VII	7

- Total the numbers.
  - 1667

5) Write 1742 as a Roman numeral.

1000	M
700	
40	
2	II

6) Write 2117 as a Roman numeral.

2000	MM
100	C
10	X
7	VII

7) Write 2019 as a Roman numeral.

2000	MM
0	
10	X
9	IX

8) Write MDCCLXXVI as a number.

M	1000
DCC	700
LXX	70
VI	6

9) Write MCDXCII as a number.

M	1000
CD	400
XC	90
II	2

10) Write MCCXV as a number.

M	1000
CC	200
X	10
V	5

Chapter 8
Scientific Notation

- **Scientific notation is an easier way to write very large and very small numbers.**
- Example: 602,200,000,000,000,000,000,000 becomes 6.022×10^{23} in scientific notation.
- Example: 0.0000000000000000019942 becomes 1.9942×10^{-18} in scientific notation.

Terminology:

- **Exponent:** The small number written just above and to the right of a base number. It is the 23 in 6.022×10^{23} and denotes the number of times 10 is used in a multiplication.
  - 10^2 denotes 10 X 10. 10^3 denotes 10 X 10 X 10.
  - A negative exponent denotes 1 divided by the 10's, which results in a number less than 1. For example, 10^{-2} is $1/10^2$, or 1/100, which is 0.01.
- **Coefficient:** The number which is multiplied by 10 raised to the exponent. It is the 6.022 in 6.022×10^{23}. It is always at least 1 and less than 10.

Steps to Write a Number in Scientific Notation

Examples using 6,154,000,000 and 0.000816:

Step 1) Separate out the digits which are either before or after all the zeros and place a decimal point after the first digit, forming the coefficient.

- 6,154,000,000:   6.154
- 0.000816:   8.16

Step 2) Look at the original number and count the number of places to move the decimal point either to the end or back to the original decimal point from the decimal point in the coefficient.

- 6,154,000,000: 9 places from between the 6 & 1 to the end.
- 0.000816: 4 places back from between the 8 & 1 to the original decimal point.

Step 3) Write the coefficient and multiply it by 10 raised to the number of places the decimal point was moved. If the decimal point was moved to the right, the exponent is positive; if the decimal point was moved to the left, the exponent is negative.

- 6.154×10^9
- 8.16×10^{-4}

Examples:

Number	Scientific Notation
5,015,000	5.015×10^6
3,000	3×10^3
645,000,000	6.45×10^8
0.00056	5.6×10^{-4}
0.00000734	7.34×10^{-6}
0.00003005	3.005×10^{-5}

Scientific Notation Exercise

1) Convert the following numbers to scientific notation.

Number	Coefficient	# of Places from New Decimal Point to end of Original Number	Coefficient X 10 Raised to the Number of Places the Decimal Point was Moved
67,000	6.7	4	6.7×10^4
8,247,000			
1,150,000			
94,800			
732,000			
921,000			
38,300,000			
2,470,000			
92,500,000			
49,230,000,000			
125,000			

2) Convert the following decimal numbers to scientific notation.

Decimal Number	Coefficient	# of Places from New Decimal Point to Original Decimal Point	Coefficient X 10 Raised to the Negative Number of Places the Decimal Point was Moved
0.056	5.6	2	5.6×10^{-2}
0.00580			
0.00070			
0.0004039			
0.005068			
0.0001332			
0.0000650			
0.00000126			
0.0000034			
0.0000783			
0.00064			

Dosage Calculations for Nursing Students-Second Edition

3) Convert the following numbers from scientific notation to numbers.

Scientific Notation	Coefficient	Exponent	# of Places to Move the Decimal Point to the Right	Number
5.62×10^6	5.62	6	6	5,620,000
7.82×10^8				
9.3×10^5				
6.2×10^7				
1.055×10^5				
2.38×10^9				
6.90×10^3				
2.781×10^8				
4.01×10^8				
7.56×10^5				

4) Convert the following decimal numbers from scientific notation to decimal numbers.

Scientific Notation	Coefficient	Exponent	# of Places to Move the Decimal Point to the Left	Decimal Number
6.05×10^{-4}	6.05	-4	4	0.000605
6.3×10^{-6}				
4.80×10^{-5}				
8.51×10^{-6}				
6.95×10^{-5}				
1.023×10^{-8}				
5.01×10^{-4}				
2.43×10^{-6}				
2.12×10^{-3}				
1.65×10^{-7}				

Unit 3: Unit Conversions

Converting within and between the various systems of measurement used in nursing is a mandatory skill. This unit also provides practice using dimensional analysis and ratio proportion, which will be valuable when moving on to dosage and IV flow rate calculations.

Chapter 9: Unit Conversions-The Basics
Summary: Covers the basic set up of unit conversion calculations using both dimensional analysis and ratio proportion. This chapter will provide a foundation for setting up dosage and IV flow rate calculations.
Importance: 10/10.

Chapter 10: Unit Conversions Within the Metric System
Summary: Covers conversions within the metric system, which are the most common in nursing.
Importance: 10/10

Chapter 11: Unit Conversions Within the Household System
Summary: Covers conversions within the household system.
Importance: 9/10

Chapter 12: Unit Conversions Between Metric, Household and Apothecary Systems
Summary: Covers conversions between all the systems.
Importance: 10/10

Chapter 13: Unit Conversions Involving Pounds and Ounces
Summary: Explains converting from pounds and ounces to pounds (e.g. 9 lb 4 oz = 9.25 lb). This is a short, easy chapter.
Importance: 8/10

Chapter 14: Unit Conversions Involving Hours and Minutes
Summary: Explains converting between hours and minutes to hours. (e.g. 3 h 30 min = 3.5 h). This is another short, easy chapter.
Importance: 8/10

Chapter 9
Unit Conversions-The Basics

Terminology:

- **Unit:** Unit of measurement. The mg, g, mL, L, oz, kg, etc., that are used in nursing calculations.
- **Unit Conversions:** Converting from one unit to another without changing the value. If you don't remember all the conversion factors, refer to the tool shed in Chapter 3.

Using the Tools in the DA Method

- Write down the quantity to be converted on the left side of the equation, say 8.67 g, and the units of the answer on the right side of the equation, say mg.

$$8.67 \text{ g} = \quad \text{mg}$$

- Look in the tool shed for the tool (conversion factor) which has mg on top and g on the bottom. Under Metric Weight you will find $\left(\frac{1000 \text{ mg}}{\text{g}}\right)$.
- Place the tool to be used next to the quantity to be converted, cancel out the units, and multiply.

$$8.67 \text{g} \left(\frac{1000 \text{ mg}}{\text{g}}\right) = 8670 \text{ mg}$$

- More than one tool may be needed to complete the conversion. For example: How many inches are there in 3.5 m?

$$3.5 \text{ m} \left(\frac{100 \text{ cm}}{\text{m}}\right) \left(\frac{1 \text{ in}}{2.54 \text{ cm}}\right) = 137.8 \text{ in}$$

Using the Tools in the RP Method

- Write a ratio with x followed by the units of the answer on top and the given on the bottom. Using the 8.67 g to mg example above:

$$\frac{x \text{ mg}}{8.67 \text{ g}}$$

- Find a ratio in the tool shed with mg on top and g on the bottom. This is the reference ratio which will be compared to the ratio containing the unknow. Place an equal sign between them.

$$\frac{x \text{ mg}}{8.67 \text{ g}} = \frac{1000 \text{ mg}}{1 \text{ g}}$$

- **Solve for x mg.** (8.67 g) (1000 mg) then divide by 1 g. x mg = 8670 mg
- If more than one tool is needed, set up another problem with the first answer as your given, or preferably, use the DA method.

Chapter 10
Unit Conversions Within the Metric System

- If needed, review Chapter 1: The Metric System
- It is highly recommended that either dimensional analysis (DA) or ratio proportion (RP) be used in these conversions.

Metric Conversion Exercise Using DA

Problem	Given to be Converted	Conversion Factor	Units of the Answer
Example	2.5 g	1000 mg/g =	2500 mg
1	340 mL	=	L
2	0.04 g	=	mg
3	25 mm	=	cm
4	2.5 dL	=	mL
5	4.5 mg	=	mcg
6	200 mcg	=	mg
7	43.5 mL	=	L
8	615 mg	=	g
9	2.5 kg	=	g
10	1.45 g	=	mg
11	3 mg	=	mcg
12	585 g	=	kg
13	75,000 mcg	=	mg
14	25 mcg	=	mg
15	3.5 L	=	mL
16	2.32 g	=	mg
17	500 mcg	=	mg
18	3 mg	=	mcg
19	25 mL	=	L
20	3.5 m	=	cm

Metric Conversion Exercise Using RP

Problem	Given	Units of the Answer	Set up Equation	Answer (Solve for x) and include units
Example	3.5 g	mg	$\dfrac{x \text{ mg}}{3.5 \text{ g}} = \dfrac{1000 \text{ mg}}{1 \text{ g}}$	3500 mg
1	5.4 g	mg		
2	354 mcg	mg		
3	5.4 kg	g		
4	102 g	kg		
5	3.5 m	cm		
6	1.6 dL	L		
7	250 mL	L		
8	4.1 g	mg		
9	25 mcg	mg		
10	6 mm	cm		
11	500 g	kg		
12	3.1 L	mL		
13	815 mcg	mg		
14	8.6 kg	g		
15	0.09 mg	mcg		

Chapter 11
Unit Conversions Within the Household System

- If needed, review Chapter 2: Apothecary/Avoirdupois/Household Systems
- It is highly recommended that either dimensional analysis (DA) or ratio proportion (RP) be used in these conversions.

Household Conversion Exercise Using DA

Problem	Given to be Converted	Conversion Factor	Units of the Answer
Example	2 fl oz	2 tbs/fl oz =	4 tbs
1	3 cups	=	fl oz
2	3 gal	=	qt
3	24 fl oz	=	cups
4	6 tsp	=	tbs
5	0.5 gal	=	pt
6	0.5 pt	=	fl oz
7	3 tsp	=	tbs
8	8 oz	=	lb
9	0.5 qt	=	fl oz
10	4 tsp	=	fl oz
11	1.5 qt	=	fl oz
12	16 fl oz	=	cups
13	4 pt	=	qt
14	6 fl oz	=	tbs
15	4 tbs	=	fl oz
16	6 tsp	=	tbs
17	2 gal	=	qt
18	3 fl oz	=	tbs
19	3 tsp	=	tbs
20	2 pt	=	fl oz

Dosage Calculations for Nursing Students-Second Edition

Household Conversion Exercise Using RP

Problem	Given	Units of the Answer	Set up Equation	Answer (Solve for x) and include units
Example	1.5 cups	fl oz	$\dfrac{x \text{ fl oz}}{1.5 \text{ cups}} = \dfrac{8 \text{ fl oz}}{1 \text{ cup}}$	12 fl oz
1	2 fl oz	tbs		
2	4 pt	gal		
3	16 fl oz	cups		
4	1.5 gal	pt		
5	3 cups	fl oz		
6	4 pt	fl oz		
7	6 tsp	tbs		
8	0.5 gal	pt		
9	3 fl oz	tbs		
10	2 tbs	fl oz		
11	3 tsp	tbs		
12	3 tbs	fl oz		
13	1.5 pt	cups		
14	2 qt	pt		
15	8 oz	lb		

Chapter 12
Unit Conversions Between Metric, Household and Apothecary Systems
- If needed, review Chapter 1: The Metric System
- If needed, review Chapter 2: Apothecary/Avoirdupois/Household Systems
- It is highly recommended that either dimensional analysis (DA) or ratio proportion (RP) be used in these conversions.

Metric, Household and Apothecary Conversion Exercise Using DA

Problem	Given to be Converted	Conversion Factor	Units of the Answer
Example	60 mL	1 fl oz/30 mL	2 fl oz
1	2 cups		mL
2	4 gr		mg
3	180 mL		fl oz
4	7 in		cm
5	0.5 pt		mL
6	98 mm		in
7	700 g		lb
8	16 in		cm
9	90 mL		fl oz
10	48 lb		kg
11	2.2 kg		lb
12	2 tbs		mL
13	1.8 fl oz		mL
14	3 gr		mg
15	60 cm		in
16	240 g		lb
17	3.2 lb		g
18	3 cups		mL
19	740 g		lb
20	65 lb		kg

Dosage Calculations for Nursing Students-Second Edition

Metric, Household and Apothecary Conversion Exercise Using RP

Problem	Given	Units of the Answer	Set up Equation	Answer (Solve for x) and include units
Example	1.5 cups	mL	$\dfrac{x \text{ mL}}{1.5 \text{ cups}} = \dfrac{240 \text{ mL}}{1 \text{ cup}}$	360 mL
1	42 kg	lb		
2	3 tbs	mL		
3	254 cm	in		
4	250 g	lb		
5	68 lb	kg		
6	10 in	cm		
7	3 gr	mg		
8	8 fl oz	pt		
9	95 mm	in		
10	750 g	lb		
11	120 mg	gr		
12	2 cups	mL		
13	15 in	cm		
14	30 mg	gr		
15	3.5 lb	oz		

Chapter 13
Unit Conversions Involving Pounds and Ounces

Occasionally, you will be given a patient's weight in pounds and ounces and will be asked to either convert it to a decimal pound amount, kilograms or grams. You will most likely find this situation in pediatric dosing problems.

Converting from Pounds and Ounces to Pounds

Example: Baby June Marie, born 12/31/18 at 1:33 PM, weighed 7 lb 4 oz. How much did she weigh in pounds?

- First, convert 4 oz to pounds. (DA will be used for these examples.)

$$4 \text{ oz} \left(\frac{1 \text{ lb}}{16 \text{ oz}}\right) = 0.25 \text{ lb}$$

- Add the whole pound quantity with the decimal pound quantity.

$$7 \text{ lb} + 0.25 \text{ lb} = 7.25 \text{ lb}$$

Converting from Pounds and Ounces to Kilograms

- First, convert pounds and ounces into pounds, then convert pounds into kg. In the above example, after 7 lb 4 oz has been converted to 7.25 lb, convert 7.25 lb to kg.

$$7.25 \text{ lb} \left(\frac{1 \text{ kg}}{2.2 \text{ lb}}\right) = 3.3 \text{ kg}$$

Converting from Pounds and Ounces to Grams

- First, convert pounds and ounces into pounds, then convert pounds into grams. In the above example, after 7 lb 4 oz has been converted to 7.25 lb, convert 7.25 lb to g.

$$7.25 \text{ lb} \left(\frac{454 \text{ g}}{\text{lb}}\right) = 3292 \text{ g}$$

Note: Follow the rounding rules of your school or facility when converting pounds and ounces to grams. Of course, since the original weight was stated to the nearest ounce, which is about 30 g, we can't be confident of the weight to the nearest gram. That being said, for problems in this section, calculate the weight to the nearest gram.

Pounds and Ounces Conversion Exercise

Convert the following to decimal pounds.

1) 8 lb 8 oz

2) 12 lb 4 oz

3) 6 lb 10 oz

4) 7 lb 9 oz

5) 5 lb 14 oz

Convert the following to kilograms.

6) 14 lb 6 oz

7) 10 lb 5 oz

8) 17 lb 9 oz

9) 16 lb 15 oz

10) 21 lb 4 oz

Convert the following to grams.

11) 3 lb 2 oz

12) 4 lb 6 oz

13) 3 lb 9 oz

14) 5 lb 7 oz

15) 5 lb 4 oz

Chapter 14
Unit Conversions Involving Hours and Minutes

Occasionally, you will be required to convert between time periods stated in decimal hours and time periods stated in hours and minutes.

An example would be converting 3.25 hours (decimal format) into 3 hours 15 minutes.

Converting from Decimal Hours to Hours and Minutes

Example: According to your calculations, an IV is scheduled to infuse for 4.3 hours. How long is that in hours and minutes?

- First, convert 0.3 hours into minutes. (DA will be used for these examples.)

$$0.3 \text{ h} \left(\frac{60 \text{ min}}{\text{h}}\right) = 18 \text{ min}$$

- Add the whole hour quantity with the minute quantity.

$$4 \text{ h} + 18 \text{ min} = 4 \text{ h } 18 \text{ min}$$

Converting from Hours and Minutes to Decimal Hours

- First, convert the minutes into hours by multiplying by (1 hour/60 min). For example, convert 3 hours 45 minutes to hours.

$$45 \text{ min} \left(\frac{1 \text{ h}}{60 \text{ min}}\right) = 0.75 \text{ h}$$

- Add the whole hours (3 h) to the decimal hours (0.75 h) resulting in 3.75 h.

Hours and Minutes Conversion Exercise

Convert the following decimal hours to hours and minutes. Round to the nearest minute.

1) 7.4 h

2) 3.8 h

3) 8.1 h

4) 10.6 h

5) 9.25 h

6) 4.5 h

7) 3.75 h

8) 12.33 h

9) 5.15 h

10) 8.2 h

Convert the following hours and minutes to decimal hours. Round to the nearest hundredth hour.

11) 8 h 43 min

12) 4 h 22 min

13) 1 h 13 min

14) 9 h 55 min

15) 8 h 10 min

16) 7 h 2 min

17) 1 h 15 min

18) 10 h 43 min

19) 8 h 40 min

20) 7 h 35 min

Unit 4: Dosage Calculations

Chapter 15: Dosage Calculations-The Basics
Summary: Covers terminology and the basic set up of dosage calculations. DA, RP and D/H x Q are explained.
Importance: 10/10.

Chapter 16: Dosage Calculations Level 1
Summary: This chapter contains practice dosage problems which are one step and require no conversion of units. If you understand simple unit conversions, these will be easy.
Importance: 10/10

Chapter 17: Dosage Calculations Level 2
Summary: This chapter covers dosage calculations which require more than one ratio. Only DA is used to explain the solutions.
Importance: 10/10

Chapter 18: Dosage Calculations Level 3
Summary: This chapter adds some twists to the problems, usually adding the patient's weight into the mix. Also, mg/kg/day type problems are covered.
Importance: 10/10

Chapter 19: Body Surface Area Dosing Calculations
Summary: The Mosteller formula to calculate BSA is explained. (Yes, sometimes you need a formula.)
Importance: 9/10

Chapter 20: Pediatric Dosage Calculations
Summary: Basic pediatric dosing calculations are covered in this chapter. The math is no different, only the type of questions asked.
Importance: 10/10

Chapter 21: Pediatric Maintenance Fluid Replacement Calculations
Summary: The formula to calculate pediatric fluid replacement is covered.
Importance: 8/10

Chapter 15
Dosage Calculations-The Basics

Terminology:

- **Dose:** The quantity of drug administered at a single time.
- **Daily dose:** The quantity of drug administered in a 24-hour period.
  - A daily dose can either be administered once daily or in divided doses and should be clarified in the order. Any ambiguity must be clarified.
- **Divided doses:** The doses which result from splitting a larger dose, usually a daily dose.
  - The details of how the divided doses are administered must be clear. For example, 150 mg per day in divided doses every 8 hours.
  - Unless otherwise stated, when daily doses are divided as follows:
    - ✓ In divided doses q 12 h means 2 equal doses per day administered every 12 hours.
    - ✓ In divided doses q 8 h means 3 equal doses per day administered every 8 hours.
    - ✓ In divided doses q 6 h means 4 equal doses per day administered every 6 hours.
    - ✓ In divided doses q 4 h means 6 equal doses per day administered every 4 hours.
  - Divided doses are not always equal and not always administered in equal time intervals. If this is the case, all the details must be included in the dosage.
- **Dosage:** The dose information along with other pertinent information relating to the frequency, duration, route of administration, etc. of the dose.
  - Example: A patient is prescribed 500 mg orally three times daily for 10 days. The dose is 500 mg; the dosage is 500 mg orally three times daily for 10 days.
- **Weight-Based Dosage:** A dosage which varies with the patient's weight.
  - Example: A patient weighing 50 kg who has been prescribed a single dose of 2 mg/kg would receive 100 mg. If the patient weighed 55 kg, he would receive 110 mg.
- **mg/kg/day:** Amount of drug in mg administered per kg of body weight each day.
  - **mg/(kg·day)** is mathematically equivalent and easier to use in calculations.
- **mcg/kg/min:** Amount of drug in mcg administered per kg of body weight each minute.
  - **mcg/(kg·min)** is mathematically equivalent and easier to use in calculations.

Step 1) Read the problem thoroughly looking for these three components:

- **The Units of the Answer:** The problem may say something like: How many mL, tablets, mg, teaspoonfuls, etc. will the patient take? Or it may say something less specific, like: What is the weight of, the volume of, how much suspension will be needed?
- **The Given of the Problem:** The problem may say something like, "A prescription is written for 10 mg, 20 mL, 1 g, etc.." or it may say, "A patient is to receive 250 mg, 5 mL, etc."
- **One or More Ratios:** All problems (other than simple unit conversions) will have a ratio somewhere in the problem; you just must learn to recognize it. It may be something like: 250 mg per 5 mL, a 50 mg tablet, 400 mcg per mL, 3 g in 100 mL. "Off the shelf" ratios may be required to complete the calculation.

Step 2) All the following problems can be solved using DA with the following equation:

- (Given) (Ratio 1) (Ratios 2, 3,...if needed) = Answer

Once the three components have been identified, the problem can be set up and solved.

Example: A patient is to receive a dose of 500 mg of amoxicillin. The pharmacy has a bottle of amoxicillin 250 mg per 5 mL suspension. How many mL of the suspension will the patient receive each dose?

- Units of the answer: mL
- The given: 500 mg
- The ratio: $\left(\frac{250 \text{ mg}}{5 \text{ mL}}\right)$

Step 3) The problem can now be set up:

- Write down the given and the units of the answer with an equal sign in between.

$$500 \text{ mg} = \text{mL}$$

- The ratio is the tool which will be used to change the units of the given (mg) into the units of the answer (mL). Remember, the ratios always equal 1 and can be flipped upside down if needed. The ratio must be placed so the units of the given are canceled out, leaving only the units of the answer. In this case, the ratio must be flipped putting mL on top and mg on the bottom.

$$500 \text{ mg} \left(\frac{5 \text{ mL}}{250 \text{ mg}}\right) = 10 \text{ mL}$$

Dealing with the Patient's Weight in DA Calculations

In a weight-based dosage, the patient's weight must be provided. For purposes of this book, the patient's weight will be the actual weight, but you should be aware that sometimes dosages are based on the ideal body weight or an adjusted body weight.

For purposes of the following examples:

- Patient weight will be in kg.
- Prescribed dose will be mg/kg.

The general setup of a DA equation is:

(Given) (Ratio 1) (Ratios 2, 3,...if needed) = Answer

Q: Where does the patient's weight go? Is it the given, a ratio, or part of the answer?
A: Technically, the patient's weight is part of the given, the other part being the amount of drug per kg (usually mg/kg).
Q: Do I start the problem with the patient's weight or the mg/kg dose?
A: You can start with either one, which is what the first edition of this book taught.
Q: Did things change for the second edition?
A: In this edition, the authors decided that it was easier to start the problem with the mg/kg dose and insert the kg weight second.

- Example: The prescriber ordered 10 mg/kg IV for your patient who weighs 75 kg. The drug is available in 10 mL vials containing 250 mg/mL. How many mL will you administer? Start by listing the mg/kg dose (the given) and the units of the answer.

$$\frac{10 \text{ mg}}{\text{kg}} = \text{mL}$$

- Now it is easy to see that mg will be changed to mL and kg will be eliminated. The job of the 75 kg weight is to eliminate kg from the equation.

$$\frac{10 \text{ mg}}{\text{kg}} \left(\frac{75 \text{ kg}}{1}\right) = \text{mL}$$

- At this point, you have the amount of drug prescribed in mg (750 mg) and only have to change mg to mL.

$$\frac{10 \text{ mg}}{\text{kg}} \left(\frac{75 \text{ kg}}{1}\right) \left(\frac{1 \text{ mL}}{250 \text{ mg}}\right) = 3 \text{ mL}$$

Q: I have seen problems where they ask how many mg/kg the patient is receiving. How do I set those up?

A: That is a common type of problem. It is also common to ask how many mg/kg/min a patient is receiving, but we will keep things simple for now.

- Example: A 50 kg patient will receive 10 mL of a drug which is available as 20 mg/mL. How many mg/kg will the patient receive? Start by listing the given (10 mL) and the units of the answer.

$$10 \text{ mL} = \frac{\text{mg}}{\text{kg}}$$

- This time mL will be changed to mg and we will add kg to the denominator of the answer. Simply insert 1/50 kg next.

$$10 \text{ mL} \left(\frac{1}{50 \text{ kg}}\right) = \frac{\text{mg}}{\text{kg}}$$

- If you stopped now, you would have 10 mL/50 kg. You only have to change the 10 mL to mg.

$$10 \text{ mL} \left(\frac{1}{50 \text{ kg}}\right)\left(\frac{20 \text{ mg}}{\text{mL}}\right) = \frac{4 \text{ mg}}{\text{kg}}$$

Q: What does all this boil down to? Try to keep it simple!

A: Use the patient's weight to either remove kg from the given or add kg into the denominator of the answer.

Using Ratio Proportion for Simple Dosage Calculations

If you have a simple dosage calculation, meaning one in which the ratio has the same units as the given and answer, you might want to use the ratio proportion method. This book doesn't recommend ratio proportion for anything other than simple unit conversions and simple dosage calculations.

Using the same example as above: A patient is to receive a dose of 500 mg of amoxicillin. The pharmacy has a bottle of amoxicillin 250 mg per 5mL suspension. How many mL of the suspension will the patient receive each dose?

- Units of the answer: mL
- The given: 500 mg
- The ratio: $\left(\frac{250 \text{ mg}}{5 \text{ mL}}\right)$

As you can see, the ratio contains the same units as the given and answer.

- Set up two ratios, one containing the given and units of the answer. The other ratio will be the ratio supplied in the problem.

$$\frac{x \text{ mL}}{500 \text{ mg}} = \frac{5 \text{ mL}}{250 \text{ mg}}$$

- Be sure to have the same units on top and bottom on both ratios.
- To solve for x: (x mL) (250 mg) = (500 mg) (5 mL)
  - x mL = ((500 mg) (5 mL))/250 mg
  - x mL = 10 mL

What about the Desired over Have x Quantity Formula?

Using the same example as above: A patient is to receive a dose of 500 mg of amoxicillin. The pharmacy has a bottle of amoxicillin 250 mg per 5 mL suspension. How many mL of the suspension will the patient receive each dose?

- The Desired is 500 mg, which in DA is the given.
- The Have is 250 mg
- The Quantity is 5 mL

The problem is set up like this:

$$\frac{500 \text{ mg}}{250 \text{ mg}} \times 5 \text{ mL} = 10 \text{ mL}$$

Compare that to the way it is set up using DA.

$$500 \text{ mg} \left(\frac{5 \text{ mL}}{250 \text{ mg}}\right) = 10 \text{ mL}$$

As you can see, in the D/H x Q, the ratio of 5 mL/250 mg is split up with the 250 mg going under the 500 mg and the 5 mL is put off to the side. If you keep the ratio together, as shown in the DA example, it is easy to add in more ratios on the more complex problems.

The authors believe that DA is superior to D/H X Q, which will not be further covered in the book.

Chapter 16
Dosage Calculations Level 1

For purposes of this book, level 1 dosage calculations are problems which are one step and require no conversion of units. The first five problems will have solutions using both DA and RP, with the remaining using DA.

Problem	Order (The Given)	Units of the Answer	Available (The Ratio)	Administer
Example (DA)	50 mg	mL	25 mg/mL	50 mg (1 mL/25 mg) = 2 mL
Example (RP)	50 mg	mL	25 mg/mL	$\dfrac{x\ mL}{50\ mg} = \dfrac{1\ mL}{25\ mg}$ x mL=2 mL
1	75 mg	mL	25 mg/mL	75 × 25 × 1 = 3 mL
2	0.3 mg	tabs	0.1 mg tabs	0.3 ÷ 0.1 3 tablets
3	75 mg	mL	150 mg/mL	75 ÷ 150 × 1 = 0.5 mL
4	8 mcg	mL	10 mcg/10 mL	8 ÷ 10 × 10 = 8 mcg (1 mcg in 1mL)
5	50 mcg	mL	100 mcg/5 mL	50 ÷ 100 × 5 = 2.5 mcg
6	0.125 mg	mL	0.25 mg/mL	0.125 ÷ 0.25 × 1 = 0.5 mg
7	150 mg	mL	300 mg/2 mL	150 ÷ 300 × 2 = 1 mg
8	7.5 mg	tabs	5 mg scored tabs	1½ tablets
9	3 mg	tabs	6 mg scored tabs	½ tablet
10	200 mcg	mL	100 mcg/mL	200 ÷ 100 × 1 = 2 mcg
11	480 mg	mL	400 mg/5 mL	480 ÷ 400 × 5 = 6 mg
12	1 g	tabs	0.25 g tab	
13	50 mcg	mL	200 mcg/mL	50 ÷ 200 × 1 = 0.25 mcg
14	0.25 mg	tabs	0.125 mg tabs	
15	1 mg	mL	10 mg/mL	1 ÷ 10 × 1 = 0.1 mg
16	90 mg	mL	60 mg/mL	90 ÷ 60 × 1 = 1.5 mg
17	150 mg	mL	100 mg/mL	150 ÷ 100 × 1 = 1.5 mg
18	40 mg	mL	50 mg/mL	40 ÷ 50 × 1 = 0.8 mg
19	0.25 g	tabs	0.5 g scored tabs	5 tablets
20	20 mg	mL	5 mg/mL	20 ÷ 5 × 1 = 4 mg

Chapter 17
Dosage Calculations Level 2

Level 2 dosage problems are a little more complex than level 1 problems and generally require more than one ratio. These problems still follow the general DA format of:

(Given) (Ratio 1) (Ratios 2, 3,..if needed) = Answer

Answers will be shown using DA only.

Example: The provider has ordered 100 mcg/day PO divided into 2 doses. You have available 0.025 mg tablets. How many tablets will you administer per dose?

You are given 100 mcg/day to start the problem and must end up with tablets/dose.

$$\frac{100 \text{ mcg}}{\text{day}} = \frac{\text{tabs}}{\text{dose}}$$

- You are required to change 100 mcg to tabs and day to dose.
- Look at the ratios provided in the problem.
  - 2 doses/day
  - 0.025 mg/tab
- You will have to supply the ratio of 1000 mcg/mg.
- Fill in the middle with the ratios so the unwanted units cancel, leaving the units of the answer.

$$\frac{100 \text{ mcg}}{\text{day}} \left(\frac{1 \text{ day}}{2 \text{ doses}}\right)\left(\frac{1 \text{ tab}}{0.025 \text{ mg}}\right)\left(\frac{1 \text{ mg}}{1000 \text{ mcg}}\right) = \frac{2 \text{ tabs}}{\text{dose}}$$

Dosage Calculations Level 2 Exercise

1) Your 42 YO patient has an order for 200 mg IM q 12 h. The drug is available as 100 mg/mL. How many mL will you administer per day?

2) The physician has ordered 1000 mg/day PO divided into 2 doses of a drug which is available in 250 mg capsules. How many capsules will you administer per dose?

3) Your patient has an order for 600 mg/day IV divided into 3 doses. You have available a 10 mL vial containing 500 mg of the drug. How many mL will you administer per dose?

4) Your pediatric patient will be going home with a 150 mL bottle of amoxicillin 125 mg/5 mL with instructions for 5 mL to be given PO q 8 h. How many days will the bottle last?

5) The NP has ordered 100 mg IM b.i.d. of a drug which is available in 5 mL vials labeled 50 mg/mL. How many mL will you administer per dose?

6) The order is 500 mcg IV. On hand you have a 2 mL vial containing 1 mg/mL. How many mL will you administer?

7) Your patient has an order for 800 mg/day IV divided into 4 doses. You have available a 5 mL vial containing 1 g of the drug. How many mL will you administer per dose?

8) Your 32 YO patient who weighs 188 lb has an order for 100 mg/day IV divided into 4 doses. The drug is available in 10 mL vials containing 50 mg/mL. How many mL will you administer per dose?

9) You have an order to administer a 400 mg dose IM of a drug which is available in 10 mL vials containing 1 g. How many mL will you administer?

10) You have an order for 0.25 mg of levothyroxine which is available in 125 mcg scored tablets. How many tablets will you administer?

Chapter 18
Dosage Calculations Level 3

Level 3 dosage problems take things up a notch from level 2 and usually incorporate the patient's weight. These problems still follow the general DA format of:

(Given) (Ratio 1) (Ratios 2, 3,..if needed) = Answer

Tip: When you see dosages expressed as mg/kg/day or mg/kg/dose, change it to mg/ (kg day) or mg/(kg dose). These forms are much easier to work with.

Answers will be shown using DA only.

Example: A 7 YO 23 kg child with acute otitis media (AOM) is to receive oral amoxicillin 80 mg/kg/day divided every 12 hours. The amoxicillin is available in 75 mL bottles containing 400 mg/5 mL. How many mL will you administer per dose?

- Look at the units of the answer first: mL/dose.
- Look at what the healthcare provider ordered: 80 mg/kg/day. This is your given and what you will start with. Remember to change 80 mg/kg/day to 80 mg/ (kg day).
- Start setting up the equation with the given and the units of the answer.

$$\frac{80 \text{ mg}}{\text{kg day}} = \frac{\text{mL}}{\text{dose}}$$

- Now you can see that you will be changing 80 mg to mL, day to dose, and eliminating kg.
- Look at the ratios provided in the problem.
  - ➤ 400 mg/5 mL
  - ➤ 2 doses/day (deduced from the dose being divided every 12 hours).
  - ➤ 75 mL/bottle (this is extra information which is irrelevant).
- To eliminate kg on the bottom, simply insert the patient's weight into the equation. If it makes it easier, enter it as 23 kg/1.
- Fill in the middle with the ratios so the unwanted units cancel, leaving the units of the answer.

$$\frac{80 \text{ mg}}{\text{kg day}} \left(\frac{23 \text{ kg}}{1}\right)\left(\frac{5 \text{ mL}}{400 \text{ mg}}\right)\left(\frac{1 \text{ day}}{2 \text{ doses}}\right) = \frac{11.5 \text{ mL}}{\text{dose}}$$

Dosage Calculations Level 3 Exercise

1) A 164 lb patient with atrial fibrillation is to receive an initial IV bolus of verapamil 0.1 mg/kg over at least 2 minutes. The drug is available in 4 mL vials containing 2.5 mg/mL. How many mL will you administer?

2) A 6 YO 46 lb child with acute otitis media (AOM) is to receive oral amoxicillin 80 mg/kg/day divided every 12 hours. The amoxicillin is available in 75 mL bottles containing 400 mg/5 mL. How many mL will you administer per dose?

3) A 4 YO 36 lb child with hypertension has be ordered furosemide 1 mg/kg/dose PO twice daily. Furosemide oral solution is available in 60 mL bottles containing 10 mg/mL. How many mL will you administer each dose?

4) A 7 YO child weighing 48 lb is diagnosed with bacterial sinusitis and is prescribed azithromycin 10 mg/kg PO once daily for 3 days. Azithromycin oral suspension is available in 15, 22.5 and 30 mL bottles containing 200 mg/5 mL. How many mL will you administer?

5) A 68 YO 173 lb patient diagnosed with an M. chelonae infection has an order for amikacin 15 mg/kg IV once daily for 2 weeks (in addition to a high dose of cefoxitin). The amikacin is available in 2 mL vials containing 500 mg. How many mL will you administer each day?

6) A 125 lb patient is to receive a single IV dose of ondansetron 0.15 mg/kg, in addition to other drugs, for prevention of chemotherapy-induced nausea and vomiting. Ondansetron is available in a 20 mL MDV of 2 mg/mL. How many mL will you administer?

7) A 74 kg male diagnosed with bacterial meningitis has an order for gentamicin 5 mg/kg/day IV in divided doses every 8 hours. How many mg will you administer for each dose?

8) Your 54 YO 162 lb, 5 ft 8 in female patient diagnosed with advanced bladder cancer has been prescribed ifosfamide 1500 mg/m²/day IV for 5 days. You calculate the BSA using the Mosteller method as being 1.88 m². Ifosfamide is available in 60 mL vials containing 3 g of drug. How many mL will you administer each day?

9) Drug abc has the following dosing guidelines:

Initiate therapy at 6-8 mg/kg/day IV once daily for 2 days, then decrease dosage by 25% for days 3 and 4, then discontinue. The prescriber has ordered an initial dose of 7 mg/kg/day IV for a 48 YO 189 lb male. The drug is available in 10 mL vials labeled 100 mg/mL.

a) How many mL will you administer on day 1?

b) How many mL will you administer on day 3? (Assume patient's weight has not changed.)

10) A 52 kg adult male diagnosed with sepsis has been prescribed IV ampicillin 150 mg/kg/day divided every 4 hours. How many mg will the patient receive each dose?

Chapter 19
Body Surface Area Dosing Calculations

Many drugs, especially chemotherapeutic drugs, are dosed by BSA (body surface area). The unit of measurement for BSA is square meter (m²). While there are several formulas to calculate BSA, this book will use the Mosteller formula:

$$BSA = \sqrt{\frac{W(kg) \times H(cm)}{3600}}$$

Where BSA is in m², W= pt weight in kg, H = pt height in cm.

Or, if using pounds and inches:

$$BSA = \sqrt{\frac{W(lb) \times H(in)}{3131}}$$

In practice, you will check with your facility on which formula to use. Also, many apps are available to quickly calculate BSA using several different formulas.

Example: Pt weight= 100 kg, height = 178 cm

$$BSA = \sqrt{\frac{100 \times 178}{3600}} = 2.22 \text{ m}^2$$

Using the same patient, but with pounds and inches:

$$BSA = \sqrt{\frac{220 \times 70}{3131}} = 2.22 \text{ m}^2$$

The formulas are the same for adults and children.

BSA Calculation Exercise

Calculate the BSA in m² for the following individuals.

1) An adult male weighing 83 kg and 185 cm tall.

2) An adult female weighing 120 lb and 5 ft 6 in tall.

3) A 13-month-old girl weighing 23 lb and 31 in tall.

4) A 16 YO female weighing 54 kg and 164 cm tall.

5) An adult male weighing 238 lb and 6 ft 6 in tall.

6) A 6 YO boy weighing 20 kg and 115 cm tall.

7) An adult male weighing 164 lb and 5 ft 9 in tall.

8) An adult female weighing 112 lb and 4 ft 10 in tall.

9) An adult male weighing 173 lb and 6 ft tall.

10) An adult female weighing 148 lb and 5 ft 1 in tall.

Calculate the following:

11) A 54 YO male patient who weighs 184 lb and is 5 ft 10 in tall is being treated for refractory multiple myeloma and will be placed on a carfilzomib 20/27 mg/m² IV twice weekly regimen. Cycle 1 of the regimen will be 20 mg/m² infused over 10 minutes on days 1 and 2, followed by 27 mg/m² over 10 minutes on days 8, 9, 15, and 16 of a 28-day treatment cycle.

a) Calculate the patient's BSA.

b) Calculate the dose in mg the patient will receive on days 1 and 2.

c) Calculate the dose the patient will receive on days 8, 9, 15, and 16.

12) A 68 YO male patient who weighs 155 lb and is 5 ft 9 in tall is being treated for acute myeloid leukemia with IV idarubicin 12 mg/m²/day for 3 days (in combination with cytarabine).

a) Calculate the patient's BSA.

b) Calculate the daily dose in mg for this patient.

13) A 10 YO 74 lb boy who is 4 ft 7 in tall is to receive IV topotecan 2.4 mg/m² once daily for 7 days for treatment of acute lymphoblastic leukemia.

a) Calculate the patient's BSA.

b) Calculate the daily dose in mg for this patient.

14) A 10 YO male child who weighs 30 kg and is 137 cm tall will start the BEACOPP regimen for treatment of Hodgkin lymphoma. Oral prednisone is part of the regimen dosed at 40 mg/m²/day in 2 divided doses on days 0 to 13.

a) Calculate the patient's BSA.

b) How many milligrams of prednisone will the patient receive per dose?

Chapter 20
Pediatric Dosage Calculations

Special care must be taken when calculating and checking pediatric dosages. Since dosages are usually based on weight or BSA, and will differ depending on the diagnosis, wide variances in dosages may exist for the same drug within the pediatric population. This makes it harder to pick out an obvious error on the prescriber's part. One area to pay special attention to is the child's charted weight. If a 15-month-old has a charted weight of 22 kg, this should raise a red flag, because unless the child is the size of a 6 or 7-year-old, someone transposed pounds and kilograms. Type in "pediatric dosing errors pounds kilograms" in your favorite search engine for more information on this problem.

A Few notes on the following problems:

- The problems in this book generally use the term "recommend dosage range" rather than "safe dosage range". Just because a dosage falls outside of the recommended range does not necessarily mean it is unsafe. Depending on the situation, it may or may not be unsafe. Any dosage falling outside of the recommended dosage should be checked with the prescriber. Of course, on your exams, if they use the term "unsafe" follow those instructions.
- The actual math in these problems is the same as adult dosage problems.
- Pay attention to rounding rules.
- Pediatric dosing problems tend to be multi-part questions. Read the entire question before beginning your calculations.
- Many pediatric dosing problems will contain a maximum dose along with a mg/kg dosing range. It is not uncommon for a prescribed dosage to fall within the recommended mg/kg range but exceed the maximum dose..

Example:

The recommended oral dosage of cephalexin to treat impetigo in infants, children and adolescents is 25 to 50 mg/kg/day divided every 6 to 8 hours (with a maximum dose of 250 mg/dose) for at least 7 days. An 18-month-old, 27 lb child has been prescribed cephalexin oral suspension 125 mg PO q 8 h for 7 days. The drug is available as 250 mg/5 mL.

Step 1) Read the dosing information thoroughly along with the four following questions. Make some mental notes.

- **The child's weight is given in pounds and the dosing is stated in mg/kg/day. You must convert pounds to kilograms.**

- A maximum dose of 250 mg is stated. Be sure to keep this in mind when answering questions 1 and 3.
- The duration of therapy is at least 7 days. Is the prescribed dosage consistent with this?

Step 2) Start the calculations.

1) What is the recommended range in mg/dose for this child when dosed q 8 h?

- You will be calculating the lowest recommended dose using 25 mg/kg/day and the highest recommended dose using 50 mg/kg/day.
- Being dosed q 8 h (every 8 hours) means 3 doses will be administered per day.

Set up the problem with your given (25 mg/kg/day) and the units of the answer (mg/dose) to calculate the low end of the recommended range. Remember to change 25 mg/kg/day to 25 mg/ (kg day).

$$\frac{25 \text{ mg}}{\text{kg day}} = \frac{\text{mg}}{\text{dose}}$$

Now you can see that you don't have to change anything on top, just eliminate kg and change day to dose.

Enter the child's weight in pounds on top along with the conversion factor for pounds to kilograms to eliminate kg in the given.

$$\frac{25 \text{ mg}}{\text{kg day}} \left(\frac{27 \text{ lb}}{1}\right)\left(\frac{1 \text{ kg}}{2.2 \text{ lb}}\right) = \frac{\text{mg}}{\text{dose}}$$

Kilograms are gone from the given. Insert the ratio of 1 day/3 doses to change day to dose.

$$\frac{25 \text{ mg}}{\text{kg day}} \left(\frac{27 \text{ lb}}{1}\right)\left(\frac{1 \text{ kg}}{2.2 \text{ lb}}\right)\left(\frac{1 \text{ day}}{3 \text{ doses}}\right) = \frac{\text{mg}}{\text{dose}}$$

Make sure the unwanted units are canceled leaving the units of the answer, mg/dose. Take out your calculator and multiply everything on top and divide by everything on the bottom.

$$\frac{25 \text{ mg}}{\text{kg day}} \left(\frac{27 \text{ lb}}{1}\right)\left(\frac{1 \text{ kg}}{2.2 \text{ lb}}\right)\left(\frac{1 \text{ day}}{3 \text{ doses}}\right) = \frac{102 \text{ mg}}{\text{dose}}$$

Substitute in 50 mg/ (kg day) to calculate the high end of the recommended range.

$$\frac{50 \text{ mg}}{\text{kg day}} \left(\frac{27 \text{ lb}}{1}\right)\left(\frac{1 \text{ kg}}{2.2 \text{ lb}}\right)\left(\frac{1 \text{ day}}{3 \text{ doses}}\right) = \frac{205 \text{ mg}}{\text{dose}}$$

Note that due to rounding, the high end of the recommended dosage is not exactly double the low end.

Answer: 102 to 205 mg/dose.

2) Is the prescribed dosage within the recommended range for impetigo?

Look at the prescribed dose and the recommended range. 125 mg/dose falls between the recommended range of 102 to 205 mg/dose.

Answer: yes

3) What is the range in mL/dose for this child?

Convert 102 mg/dose and 205 mg/dose to mL/dose. You will use the ratio 250 mg/5 mL, which will be flipped upside down.

$$\frac{102 \text{ mg}}{\text{dose}} \left(\frac{5 \text{ mL}}{250 \text{ mg}} \right) = \frac{2.04 \text{ mL}}{\text{dose}}$$

This would be rounded to the nearest tenth mL, which is 2.0 mL/dose, but you drop the trailing zero for safety reasons, leaving 2 mL/dose.

$$\frac{205 \text{ mg}}{\text{dose}} \left(\frac{5 \text{ mL}}{250 \text{ mg}} \right) = \frac{4.1 \text{ mL}}{\text{dose}}$$

Answer: 2 to 4.1 mL/dose.

4) How many mL/dose would the child receive for the prescribed dosage?

Look back at the prescribed dosage, 125 mg PO q 8 h for 7 days. 125 mg is the amount per dose.

$$\frac{125 \text{ mg}}{\text{dose}} \left(\frac{5 \text{ mL}}{250 \text{ mg}} \right) = \frac{2.5 \text{ mL}}{\text{dose}}$$

Do you tell the mom (or dad) just to give one-half teaspoonful measured with a kitchen teaspoonful? NO! Make sure they use a measuring device calibrated in milliliters.

Pediatric Dosage Calculations Exercise

1) The recommended oral dosage of penicillin V potassium (penicillin VK) to treat community acquired pneumonia (CAP) in infants, children and adolescents is 50 to 75 mg/kg/day in 3 to 4 divided doses (with a maximum daily dose of 2000 mg) for 7-10 days. A 4 YO 36 lb child has been prescribed penicillin VK oral solution 250 mg PO q.i.d. for 10 days. The drug is available as 250 mg/5 mL.

1) What is the recommended range in mg/dose for this child when dosed q.i.d. (4 times daily)?

2) Is the prescribed dosage within the recommended range for CAP?

3) What is the range in mL/dose for this child?

4) How many mL/dose would the child receive for the prescribed dosage?

The recommended oral dosage of cephalexin to treat community acquired pneumonia caused by S. aureus (methicillin-susceptible) in children and adolescents is 75 to 100 mg/kg/day in 3 to 4 divided doses (with a maximum daily dose of 4000 mg/day) for 7-10 days. A 4 YO child weighing 34 lb has been prescribed 500 mg PO q 8 h for 7 days. The drug is available as 250 mg/5 mL.

5) What is the recommended range in mg/dose for this child when dosed q 8 h?

6) Is the prescribed dosage within the recommended range for this diagnosis?

7) What is the range in mL/dose for this child?

8) How many mL/dose would the child receive for the prescribed dosage?

The recommended oral dosage for diphenhydramine is 5 mg/kg/day divided into 3-4 doses, with a maximum daily dose of 300 mg/day, when treating allergies in infants, children and adolescents. An 8 YO 57 lb male child has been prescribed 30 mg PO q 6 h. Diphenhydramine is available as an oral solution containing 12.5 mg/5 mL.

9) Is this a reasonable dosage for this child?

10) How many mL/dose will the child receive?

The dosing guidelines for oral morphine sulfate solution for treating moderate to severe acute pain in infants >6 months, children and adolescents who are <50 kg is 0.2 to 0.5 mg/kg/dose every 3 to 4 hours as needed and for children and adolescents 50 kg and over it is 15 to 20 mg every 3 to 4 hours as needed. Morphine sulfate oral solution 2 mg/mL and 4 mg/mL is available.

11) Using the above information, what is the normal mg/dose range for a 10 YO 32 kg male child?

12) What is the normal mL/dose range using the 2 mg/mL solution for a 13-month-old 20 lb child?

13) The prescriber has ordered 2 mL/dose of the 4 mg/mL morphine sulfate solution for your 4 YO patient who weighs 18 kg. Is this dose within the dosing guidelines?

14) The prescriber, who wants to order the highest recommended dose of oral morphine sulfate solution for a 14 kg 3 YO child, has ordered 3.9 mL of the 4 mg/mL solution. Is this the correct dose? If not, what is a possible cause of the error?

Chapter 21
Pediatric Maintenance Fluid Replacement Calculations

Weight	24 Hour Fluid Requirement
Infants 3.5 to 10 kg	100 mL/kg
Children 11-20 kg	1000 mL + 50 mL/kg for every kg over 10
For children > 20 kg	1500 mL + 20 mL/kg for every kg over 20, up to a maximum of 2400 mL daily.

Use the above table in the following calculations. Round to the nearest mL and nearest mL/h.

Example: Calculate the daily maintenance fluid requirement for an NPO (nothing by mouth) child weighing 14 kg.

1000 mL + 4 kg (50 mL/kg) = 1000 mL + 200 mL = 1200 mL

At what rate would you set the infusion pump?

1200 mL/24 h = 50 mL/h

Pediatric Maintenance Fluid Replacement Calculations Exercise

1) Calculate the daily maintenance fluid requirement for an NPO child weighing 42.5 kg.

2) Calculate the daily maintenance fluid requirement for an NPO child weighing 24 kg.

3) Calculate the daily maintenance fluid requirement for an NPO child weighing 13 kg.

4) Calculate the daily maintenance fluid requirement for an NPO child weighing 9.5 kg.

5) A 37 kg NPO child is on 70% fluid maintenance (70% of the calculated amount in the above table). At what rate will you set the infusion pump?

6) What is the daily maintenance fluid requirement for an NPO child on 70% fluid maintenance who weighs 17.5 kg? At what rate will you set the infusion pump?

7) What is the daily maintenance fluid requirement for an NPO child on 70% fluid maintenance who weighs 34 kg?

8) Calculate the daily maintenance fluid requirement for an NPO child weighing 30.5 kg.

9) Calculate the infusion rate to deliver daily maintenance fluids to an NPO child weighing 36 kg.

10) What is the daily maintenance fluid requirement for an NPO child on 70% fluid maintenance who weighs 43 kg? At what rate will you set the infusion pump?

11) At what rate will you set the infusion pump to deliver maintenance fluids to a 17 kg NPO child who is on 70% fluid maintenance?

12) Calculate the daily maintenance fluid requirement for an NPO child weighing 29 kg.

Unit 5: IV Flow Rate Calculations

Chapter 22: IV Flow Rate Calculations-The Basics
Summary: The terminology and basic set up of the three main types of IV flow rate calculations is covered in this chapter.
Importance: 10/10.

Chapter 23: IV Flow Rate Calculations Level 1
Summary: Simple, one step, calculations involving the three main types of IV flow rate problems are covered in this chapter.
Importance: 10/10

Chapter 24: IV Flow Rate Calculations Level 2
Summary: Chapter 24 covers more complex IV flow rate problems, which may include the patient's weight, mcg/kg/min type rates, and unnecessary information. These problems still follow the same general set up of level 1 problems.
Importance: 10/10

Chapter 25: IV Flow Rate Adjustments
Summary: This chapter covers the procedure to adjust an IV flow rate when the initial set rate has not been infusing correctly.
Importance: 10/10

Chapter 26: Heparin Infusion and Adjustment Calculations
Summary: This chapter will test your ability to follow directions regarding heparin infusions. The actual math is the same, but you must pay attention to dose rounding, maximum dose, and adjustment instructions. Fun stuff!
Importance: 9/10

Chapter 22
IV Flow Rate Calculations-The Basics

Terminology:

- **IV:** Abbreviation for intravenous, meaning administered into a vein.
- **drop factor:** The number of drops (gtts) per mL. Macrodrip tubing comes 10, 15, 20 gtts/mL while microdrip tubing is 60 gtts/mL.
- **VTBI:** Volume to be infused.
- **flow rate/infusion rate/drip rate:** The volume of solution or weight of drug delivered over time. The units are usually gtts/min, mL/hour or mg/hour.

These problems are solved in the same manner as unit conversion and dosage problems. There is a given, units of the answer, and one or more ratios which will be used to convert the units of the given into the units of the answer.

The general setup of an IV flow rate problem is:

(Given)(Ratios) = Answer

The problem will supply you with the given and the units of the answer. The ratios will either be supplied in the problem, or you may have to use your own (60 min/h, 1000 mcg/mg, etc.).

There are three main types of IV Flow rate problems:

- The **rate to rate** problem is the most common. For example: An IV is running at a rate of 1 liter per hour with a drop factor of 20 (20 drops/mL). What is the rate in drops/min?
  If the units of the answer are a rate, the given must be a rate.

(Rate)(Ratios) = Rate

- The **time to quantity** problem will give you a time duration and ask for the quantity of something (mL, mg, mg/kg, mEq) delivered over that duration. For example: An IV with a flow rate of 500 mL/h has been running for 2 hours. What volume of fluid has been administered?
  If the units of the answer are a quantity, the given must be a time duration.

(Time)(Ratios) = Quantity

- The **quantity to time** is just the opposite of the time to quantity problem. You will be given a quantity of something and asked for the time duration to administer it. For example: How long will it take to administer 1 L of fluid at the rate of 250 mL/h?
  If the units of the answer are a time duration, the given must be a quantity.

(Quantity)(Ratios) = Time

Examples:

1) 1000 mL is infused over 4 hours using an infusion set with a drop factor of 10 (10 gtts/mL). Calculate the flow rate in gtts/min.

Step 1) Look at the units of the answer. Gtts/min is a rate, so the given must be a rate. The only other rate in the problem is 1000 mL/4 h. Write these down with an equal sign.

$$\frac{1000 \text{ mL}}{4 \text{ h}} = \frac{\text{gtts}}{\text{min}}$$

Now you can see that you have to change mL to gtts and h to min. The ratio of $\frac{10 \text{ gtts}}{\text{mL}}$ will change mL to gtts and the ratio $\frac{1 \text{ h}}{60 \text{ min}}$ will change hours to minutes.

Step 2) Arrange the ratios so the unwanted units cancel leaving the units of the answer.

$$\frac{1000 \text{ mL}}{4 \text{ h}} \left(\frac{10 \text{ gtts}}{\text{mL}}\right) \left(\frac{1 \text{ h}}{60 \text{ min}}\right) = \frac{\text{gtts}}{\text{min}}$$

Step 3) Take out your calculator and do the calculations. Multiply everything on top and divide by everything on the bottom, giving the answer of 41.7 gtts/min which is rounded to 42 gtts/min.

$$\frac{1000 \text{ mL}}{4 \text{ h}} \left(\frac{10 \text{ gtts}}{\text{mL}}\right) \left(\frac{1 \text{ h}}{60 \text{ min}}\right) = \frac{42 \text{ gtts}}{\text{min}}$$

2) A patient has an order for regular insulin at the rate of 18 units/hour. The solution is 100 mL with 100 units of regular insulin. An infusion set with a drop factor of 20 is being used. What will be the flow rate in gtts/min?

Step 1) Looking at the units of the answer you see gtts/min, so you know the given must be a rate. The only other rate in the problem is 18 units/hour, so you know this is the given.

$$\frac{18 \text{ units}}{\text{h}} = \frac{\text{gtts}}{\text{min}}$$

You will have to change units to gtts and hours to minutes. It will take two ratios to change units to gtts, $\frac{100 \text{ mL}}{100 \text{ units}}$ and $\frac{20 \text{ gtts}}{\text{mL}}$. The ratio of $\frac{1 \text{ h}}{60 \text{ min}}$ will change hours to minutes.

Step 2) Arrange the ratios so the unwanted units cancel leaving the units of the answer. Double check everything and do the calculations.

$$\frac{18 \text{ units}}{\text{h}} \left(\frac{100 \text{ mL}}{100 \text{ units}}\right) \left(\frac{20 \text{ gtts}}{\text{mL}}\right) \left(\frac{1 \text{ h}}{60 \text{ min}}\right) = \frac{6 \text{ gtts}}{\text{min}}$$

3) A patient has an order for a drug to be infused at the rate of 25 mg/kg/h. A 1 L bag contains 10 g of the drug and the patient weighs 80 kg. An infusion set with a drop factor of 15 is being used. What is the flow rate in gtts/min?

This problem looks a little different because it contains the rate 25 mg/kg/h. This means (25 mg/kg)/h. You can either enter the rate as $\frac{25 \text{ mg/kg}}{h}$ or our prefered way $\frac{25 \text{ mg}}{kg \; h}$, which is mathematically equivalent.

Step 1) Look at the units of the answer. gtts/min is a rate, so the given must be a rate. The only other rate in the problem is 25 mg/kg/h. Write these down with an equal sign.

$$\frac{25 \text{ mg}}{kg \; h} = \frac{gtts}{min}$$

You will have to change mg to gtts and h to minutes. kg is not changed to anything, but rather eliminated from the equation. The patient's weight is part of the given and will be inserted above the line to eliminate kg.

Step 2) Arrange the ratios and the patient's weight so the unwanted units cancel leaving the units of the answer. Double check everything and do the calculations.

$$\frac{25 \; \cancel{mg}}{\cancel{kg} \; \cancel{h}} \left(\frac{80 \; \cancel{kg}}{1}\right)\left(\frac{1\cancel{L}}{10 \; \cancel{g}}\right)\left(\frac{1 \; \cancel{g}}{1000 \; \cancel{mg}}\right)\left(\frac{1000 \; \cancel{mL}}{\cancel{L}}\right)\left(\frac{15 \; gtts}{\cancel{mL}}\right)\left(\frac{1 \; \cancel{h}}{60 \; min}\right) = \frac{50 \; gtts}{min}$$

4) Calculate the length of time required to infuse a 1000 mL bag at the rate of 50 mL/h.

Step 1) Look at the units of the answer. Although it doesn't say "Calculate the number of hours", you can figure that out yourself. Since the units of the answer is a time duration, you know that the given must be a quantity. The only quantity in the problem is 1000 mL.

$$1000 \text{ mL} = \text{hours}$$

Step 2) Whenever you have a time to quantity or quantity to time problem, one of the ratios must be a rate. The only rate in the problem is 50 mL/h, so you know that must be part of the equation.

$$1000 \; \cancel{mL} \left(\frac{1 \; h}{50 \; \cancel{mL}}\right) = 20 \; h$$

5) An IV has been running for 2 hours at the rate of 40 mL/h. How many mL have been administered?

This is an example of a simple time to quantity problem. The units of the answer are mL, so the given must be a time duration.

$$2 \text{ h} = \text{mL}$$

The rate of 40 mL/h will change h to mL.

$$2\cancel{\text{h}}\left(\frac{40 \text{ mL}}{\cancel{\text{h}}}\right) = 80 \text{ mL}$$

Summary

1) Look at the units of the answer.

- If it is a rate, the given will be a rate.
- If it is a duration of time, the given will be a quantity.
- If it is a quantity, the given will be a duration of time.

2) Compare the given to the units of the answer.

3) Insert the ratios so the unwanted units cancel leaving the units of the answer.

4) Double check everything and do the calculations.

Chapter 23
IV Flow Rate Calculations Level 1

These are the most basic IV flow rate problems and involve calculating the flow rates in either mL/h, if using an infusion pump, or drops/minute, if using gravity infusion. Refer to Chapter 20 for specifics on setting up the problems.

Round all drops/min to the nearest drop. Round all mL/hour rates for the infusion pump to the nearest tenth mL/hour.

Calculate the flow rate in mL/h.

1) 1000 mL infused over 5 hours.

2) 500 mL infused over 7 hours 30 minutes.

3) 500 mL infused over 5 hours 30 minutes.

4) 1000 mL infused over 8 hours.

5) 250 mL infused over 45 minutes.

Calculate the flow rate in drops/min.

6) 1000 mL infused over 10 hours 30 minutes with a drop factor of 60 (60 gtts/mL).

7) 500 mL infused over 90 minutes with a drop factor of 10.

8) 1000 mL infused over 5 hours with a drop factor of 15.

9) 250 mL infused over 2 hours with a microdrip set (60 gtts/mL).

10) 500 mL infused over 4 hours 15 minutes with a drop factor of 20.

Calculate the length of time in hours and minutes, rounded to the nearest minute, required to infuse the following:

11) 1000 mL at 63 mL/h.

12) 250 mL at 30 gtts/min with a drop factor of 20.

13) 1000 mL at 80 mL/h.

14) 1000 mL at 50 gtts/min with a drop factor of 10.

15) 500 mL at 43 gtts/min with a drop factor of 10.

Calculate the volume infused in the following scenarios. Round to the nearest mL.

16) Infusion rate of 60 mL per hour for 1 hour 15 min.

17) Infusion rate of 38 mL/h for 90 min.

18) Infusion rate of 67 mL/h for 2 hours 30 min.

19) Infusion rate of 40 gtts/min, drop factor 20, for 6 hours 45 min.

20) Infusion rate of 28 gtts/min, drop factor 20, for 4 hours 30 min.

Chapter 24
IV Flow Rate Calculations Level 2

These problems are a step up from the basic problems and generally involve the patient's weight. Refer to Chapter 21 for specifics on setting up the problems. Remember, if you see something like mcg/kg/min, change it to mcg/(kg min).

Round all drops/min to the nearest drop. Round all mL/hour rates for the infusion pump to the nearest tenth mL/hour.

1) Mrs. Wilson, who has been diagnosed with acute decompensated heart failure, has an order for nitroglycerin 10 mcg/min IV. Mrs. Wilson weighs 131 lb. The NTG is available as 100 mg/250 mL. At what rate will you set the IV infusion pump?

2) A 42 YO female who weighs 78 kg is to receive vancomycin 2 g in 400 mL D5W at a rate of 10 mg/min. At what rate will you set the IV infusion pump?

3) Your 61 YO 72 kg patient has an order for a lidocaine infusion at the rate of 20 mcg/kg/min. You have a 250 mL bag labeled "Lidocaine HCl and 5% Dextrose Injection USP". Lidocaine 2 g (8 mg/mL) is printed in big red letters in the middle of the label. What rate will you set the IV infusion pump?

4) A healthcare provider has ordered dobutamine 10 mcg/kg/min IV for your 65 YO patient who weighs 165 lb. The dobutamine is available as 1000 mg/250 mL. At what rate will you set the IV infusion pump?

5) Your 68 kg patient is receiving a dopamine infusion at the rate of 14 mL/h. The dopamine is mixed as 200 mg of dopamine in 250 mL of D5W. The infusion has been running for 1 hour 45 minutes. How many mcg/kg/min is the patient receiving

6) A 37 YO female weighing 118 lb, who is being treated for a bite wound infection, has an order for ciprofloxacin 400 mg IV every 12 hours to be infused by slow IV infusion over 60 minutes. Ciprofloxacin is available in 200 mL bags containing 400 mg. You are using an IV administration set with a drop factor of 20. How many drops/min will you administer?

7) A 160 lb patient has an order for dopamine 15 mcg/kg/min to treat heart failure. The courteous pharmacy staff sends a 250 mL bag labeled dopamine 3200 mcg/mL. At what rate will you set the IV infusion pump?

8) Your 186 lb patient in vasodilatory shock has been ordered vasopressin 0.03 units/min IV. The vasopressin is available as 20 units/100 mL. At what rate will you set the IV infusion pump?

9) A 57 YO male weighing 72 kg, who has been diagnosed with meningitis, has an order for gentamicin 5 mg/kg/day in 3 divided doses. Each dose is to be administered over 120 minutes. The drug is available in 100 mL bags containing 125 mg. At what rate will you set the IV infusion pump?

10) Your 53 kg patient is experiencing angina and has been titrated up from a starting dose of 5 mcg/min to 20 mcg/min of IV nitroglycerin. The NTG is available as 100 mg/250 mL. At what rate will you set the IV infusion pump?

11) A 24 lb, 11-month-old infant, in shock has an order for norepinephrine 0.1 mcg/kg/min IV. The norepinephrine is available in a concentration of 8 mcg/mL. At what rate will you set the IV infusion pump?

12) Your 57 YO female patient, who has been diagnosed with septic shock, weighs 165 lb. She has an order for norepinephrine 0.1 mcg/kg/min IV. The pharmacy delivers a bag containing 4 mg norepinephrine in 250 mL D5NS. At what rate will you set the IV infusion pump?

13) Your 162 lb patient in vasodilatory shock has had his vasopressin titrated up to 0.035 units/min IV. The vasopressin is available as 20 units/100 mL. What rate will you set the IV infusion pump?

14) Your 66 kg patient in septic shock has been ordered norepinephrine 1.5 mcg/kg/min IV. The norepinephrine is available as 4 mg in 250 mL D5W. What rate will you set the IV infusion pump?

15) A 50 YO male weighing 62 kg is to receive tobramycin 2 mg/kg/dose IV every 8 hours for a severe infection. Each dose will be administered over 40 minutes.

a) How many mg will the patient receive each dose?

b) The pharmacy sends over the appropriate dose of tobramycin in a 100 mL bag of NS. At what rate will you set the IV infusion pump?

16) A patient who weighs 165 lb is suffering from acute hypertension and has an order to start an infusion of nitroprusside 0.4 mcg/kg/min. The pharmacy delivers a 1000 mL bag containing 50 mg nitroprusside in D5W. At what rate will you set the IV infusion pump?

17) Your 91 kg patient is receiving a dopamine infusion at the rate of 15 mL/h. The dopamine is mixed as 200 mg of dopamine in 250 mL of D5W. The infusion has been running for 1 hour 25 minutes. How many mcg/kg/min is the patient receiving?

18) A 9 kg, 10-month-old infant, in shock has an order for norepinephrine 0.05 mcg/kg/min IV. The norepinephrine is available in a concentration of 8 mcg/mL. At what rate will you set the IV infusion pump?

19) Your 51 kg 62 YO patient diagnosed with bradycardia has an order for epinephrine 0.3 mcg/kg/min. The efficient pharmacy sends over a bag containing 1 mg epinephrine in 250 mL D5W. At what rate will you set the IV infusion pump?

20) R.M, a 69 YO female weighing 67 kg with heart failure, has an order for a continuous IV infusion of milrinone 0.5 mcg/kg/min. Milrinone is available in 100 mL bags containing 20 mg. At what rate will you set the IV infusion pump?

Chapter 25
IV Flow Rate Adjustments

Occasionally, you will be required to adjust the flow rate of an IV which hasn't been infusing at the desired rate. For example, you may have an order to infuse a 1000 mL bag over 8 hours, but after 4 hours you notice that 600 mL remain, meaning that only 400 mL has infused, rather than the desired 500 mL. You must now recalculate the flow rate so that the remaining 600 mL infuses over 4 hours. Depending on facility policy, you may have to contact the prescriber if a significant adjustment has been made. For purposes of these problems, assume the prescriber must be contacted for any flow rate change of 25% or more.

Example: A 1000 mL bag of D5W was started at 0900 and set to infuse over 6 hours with a drop factor of 20. At 1100 you monitor the infusion and notice that 800 mL remains.

What is the initial calculated rate in gtts/min?

$$\frac{1000 \text{ mL}}{6 \text{ h}} \left(\frac{20 \text{ gtts}}{\text{mL}}\right)\left(\frac{1 \text{ h}}{60 \text{ min}}\right) = \frac{56 \text{ gtts}}{\text{min}}$$

What will be the new rate in gtts/min?

You will infuse the remaining 800 mL over 4 hours using the same drop set.

$$\frac{800 \text{ mL}}{4 \text{ h}} \left(\frac{20 \text{ gtt}}{\text{mL}}\right)\left(\frac{1 \text{ h}}{60 \text{ min}}\right) = \frac{67 \text{ gtts}}{\text{min}}$$

What is the percent change?

The formula to calculate percent change is:

$$\frac{\text{Final} - \text{Initial}}{\text{Initial}} (100\%) = \% \text{ Change}$$

All the units will cancel, so we can just use 67 and 56, rather than 67 gtts/min and 56 gtts/min.

$$\frac{67 - 56}{56} (100\%) = 19.6\,\%$$

Will you contact the prescriber?

No, 19.6% is <25%.

IV Flow Rate Adjustments Exercise

You have an order for a 500 mL bag of NS to infuse over 4 hours 30 minutes with a drop factor of 15. The bag was started at 1800. At 1900 you notice that 300 mL remain.

1) What is the initial calculated rate in gtts/min?

2) What will be the new rate in gtts/min?

3) What is the percent change?

4) Will you contact the prescriber?

You have an order for a 1000 mL bag of NS to infuse over 4 hours with a drop factor of 20. The bag was started at 0800. At 0900 you notice that 850 mL remain.

5) What is the initial calculated rate in gtts/min?

6) What will be the new rate in gtts/min?

7) What is the percent change?

8) Will you contact the prescriber?

You have an order for a 1000 mL bag of D5W to infuse over 9 hours with a drop factor of 20. The bag was started at 0800. At 1400 you notice that 400 mL remain.

9) What is the initial calculated rate in gtts/min?

10) What will be the new rate in gtts/min?

88 | Page

Dosage Calculations for Nursing Students-Second Edition

11) What is the percent change?

12) Will you contact the prescriber?

You have an order for a 500 mL bag of NS to infuse over 2 hours with a drop factor of 20. The bag was started at 1000. At 1030 you notice that 400 mL remain.

13) What is the initial calculated rate in gtts/min?

14) What will be the new rate in gtts/min?

15) What is the percent change?

16) Will you contact the prescriber?

You have an order for a 250 mL bag of NS to infuse over 2 hours with a drop factor of 60. The bag was started at 1900. At 1930 you notice that 175 mL remain.

17) What is the initial calculated rate in gtts/min?

18) What will be the new rate in gtts/min?

19) What is the percent change?

20) Will you contact the prescriber?

Chapter 26
Heparin Infusion and Adjustment Calculations

Heparin is an anticoagulant used to treat various conditions including heart attacks, deep vein thrombosis, atrial fibrillation, and pulmonary embolism. Heparin infusion protocols vary by facility, so these practice problems will probably differ from your actual calculations. The key to these problems is paying attention to the instructions.

For this set of problems, use the following information:

- Round bolus doses to the nearest 500 units.
- Round infusion doses to the nearest 100 units/h.
- Use 25,000 units heparin/250 mL D5W (100 units/mL) for infusions.
- Use 5000 units/mL for IVP bolus calculations.
- Heparin levels are monitored by anti-Xa assay 6 hours after starting the infusion and 6 hours after each dosage adjustment.
- After two consecutive anti-Xa levels are within therapeutic range (0.3-0.7 units/mL) decrease to daily monitoring.
- Contact prescriber if two consecutive anti-Xa levels are > 0.9 or < 0.2.
- Use the following table for dosage adjustments.

Anti-Xa (units/mL)	Re-Bolus	Hold Infusion	Dosage Adjustment
< 0.2	80 units/kg	No	Increase 4 units/kg/h
0.2-0.29	40 units/kg	No	Increase 2 units/kg/h
0.3-0.7	No	No	No Change
0.71-0.8	No	No	Decrease 1 unit/kg/h
0.81-0.9	No	30 min	Decrease 2 units/kg/h
>0.9	No	60 min	Decrease 3 units/kg/h

Example:

Pt L.W, who weighs 182 lb, has been admitted with a diagnosis of DVT and has the following heparin order:
Initial bolus: 80 units/kg (max 10,000 units)
Initial infusion: 18 units/kg/h (initial max of 1800 units/h)

a) Calculate the bolus dose in units.

$$\frac{80 \text{ units}}{\text{kg}} \left(\frac{182 \text{ lb}}{1}\right)\left(\frac{1 \text{ kg}}{2.2 \text{ lb}}\right) = 6618 \text{ units rounded to } 6500 \text{ units}$$

b) Calculate the bolus dose in mL.

$$6500 \text{ units}\left(\frac{1 \text{ mL}}{5000 \text{ units}}\right) = 1.3 \text{ mL}$$

c) Calculate the initial infusion rate in units/h.

$$\frac{18 \text{ units}}{\text{kg h}} \left(\frac{182 \text{ lb}}{1}\right)\left(\frac{1 \text{ kg}}{2.2 \text{ lb}}\right) = \frac{1489 \text{ units}}{\text{h}} \text{ rounded to } \frac{1500 \text{ units}}{\text{h}}$$

d) Calculate the initial infusion rate in mL/h.

$$\frac{1500 \text{ units}}{\text{h}} \left(\frac{1 \text{ mL}}{100 \text{ units}}\right) = \frac{15 \text{ mL}}{\text{h}}$$

e) The initial infusion was started at 1300. At 1900 you order an anti-Xa assay and it comes back at 0.75 units/mL. What will the new infusion rate be in units/h?

Decrease by 1 unit/kg/h resulting in new rate of 17 units/kg/h.

$$\frac{17 \text{ units}}{\text{kg h}} \left(\frac{182 \text{ lb}}{1}\right)\left(\frac{1 \text{ kg}}{2.2 \text{ lb}}\right) = \frac{1406 \text{ units}}{\text{h}} \text{ rounded to } \frac{1400 \text{ units}}{\text{h}}$$

f) At 0100 the following day another anti-Xa assay is ordered and comes back at 0.69 units/mL. Will you, or the on-duty nurse, adjust the dose? If so, what will the new infusion rate be in units/h?

No dosage adjustment.

g) At 0700 another anti-Xa assay is ordered which comes back at 0.70 units/mL. What is your course of action?

No dosage adjustment and decrease to daily monitoring.

Heparin Infusion and Adjustment Calculations Exercise

Pt C.B, a 55 YO female weighing 165 lb, has been admitted with a diagnosis of PE and has the following heparin order:
Initial bolus: 80 units/kg (max 10,000 units)
Initial infusion: 18 units/kg/h (initial max of 1800 units/h)

1) Calculate the bolus dose in units.

2) Calculate the bolus dose in mL.

3) Calculate the initial infusion rate in units/h.

4) Calculate the initial infusion rate in mL/h.

5) The initial infusion was started at 0630. At 12:30 PM you order an anti-Xa assay and it comes back at 0.95 units/mL.

a) What course of action will you take?

b) What will the new infusion rate be in units/h?

6) At 1830 another anti-Xa assay is ordered and comes back at 0.91 units/mL. What is your course of action?

7) After contacting the prescriber after the second anti-Xa assay >9.0, you are instructed to decrease the dosage by 3 units/kg/h. What will be the new rate in units/h?

Pt Y.M, who weighs 174 lb, has been admitted with a diagnosis of unstable angina and has the following heparin order:
Initial bolus: 60 units/kg (max 5,000 units)
Initial infusion: 12 units/kg/h (initial max of 1000 units/h)

8) Calculate the bolus dose in units.

9) Calculate the bolus dose in mL.

10) Calculate the initial infusion rate in units/h.

11) Calculate the initial infusion rate in mL/h.

12) The initial infusion was started at 1600. At 2200 you order an anti-Xa assay and it comes back at 0.24 units/mL.

a) What course of action will you take?

b) Include all calculations.

13) At 0400 the following day another anti-Xa assay is ordered and comes back at 0.51 units/mL. Will you, or the on-duty nurse, adjust the dose? If so, what will the new infusion rate be in units/h?

14) At 1000 another anti-Xa assay is ordered which comes back at 0.72 units/mL.

a) What is your course of action?

b) Include all calculations.

Pt T.G., who weighs 84 kg, has been admitted with a diagnosis of DVT and has the following heparin order:
Initial bolus: 80 units/kg (max 10,000 units)
Initial infusion: 18 units/kg/h (initial max of 1800 units/h)

15) Calculate the bolus dose in units.

16) Calculate the bolus dose in mL.

17) Calculate the initial infusion rate in units/h.

18) Calculate the initial infusion rate in mL/h.

19) The initial infusion was started at 1300. At 1900 you order an anti-Xa assay and it comes back at 0.77 units/mL.

a) What course of action will you take?

b) Include all calculations.

20) At 0100 the following day another anti-Xa assay is ordered and comes back at 0.69 units/mL. Will you, or the on-duty nurse, adjust the dose? If so, what will the new infusion rate be in units/h?

21) At 0700 another anti-Xa assay is ordered which comes back at 0.70 units/mL.

a) What is your course of action?

b) Include all calculations.

Pt D.E, who weighs 79 kg, has been admitted with a diagnosis of stroke and has the following heparin order:

Initial bolus: None

Initial infusion: 12 units/kg/h (initial max of 1200 units/h)

22) Calculate the bolus dose in units.

23) Calculate the bolus dose in mL.

24) Calculate the initial infusion rate in units/h.

25) Calculate the initial infusion rate in mL/h.

26) The initial infusion was started at 9:30 AM. At 3:30 PM you order an anti-Xa assay and it comes back at 0.55 units/mL.

a) What is your course of action?

b) Include all calculations.

27) At 9:30 PM another anti-Xa assay is ordered and comes back at 0.51 units/mL.

a) Will you, or the on-duty nurse, adjust the dose?

b) If so, what will the new infusion rate be in mL/h?

28) At 0700 another anti-Xa assay is ordered which comes back at 0.53 units/mL.

a) What is your course of action?

b) When will you order the next anti-Xa?

Pt B.B., who weighs 49 kg, has been admitted with a diagnosis of PE and has the following heparin order:
Initial bolus: 80 units/kg (max 10,000 units)
Initial infusion: 18 units/kg/h (initial max of 1800 units/h)

29) Calculate the bolus dose in units.

30) Calculate the bolus dose in mL.

31) Calculate the initial infusion rate in units/h.

32) Calculate the initial infusion rate in mL/h.

33) The initial infusion was started at 1000. At 1600 you order an anti-Xa assay and it comes back at 0.26 units/mL.

a) What course of action do you take?

b) Include all calculations.

34) At 2200 another anti-Xa assay is ordered and comes back at 0.40 units/mL.

a) Will you, or the on-duty nurse, adjust the dose?

b) If so, what will the new infusion rate be in units/h?

35) At 0400 the next day, another anti-Xa assay is ordered which comes back at 0.42 units/mL. What is your course of action?

Pt P.J., a 68 YO male weighing 83 kg has been admitted with a diagnosis of unstable angina and has the following heparin order:
Initial bolus: 60 units/kg (max 5,000 units)
Initial infusion: 12 units/kg/h (initial max of 1000 units/h)

36) Calculate the bolus dose in units.

37) Calculate the bolus dose in mL.

38) Calculate the initial infusion rate in units/h.

39) Calculate the initial infusion rate in mL/h.

40) The initial infusion was started at 1600. At 2200 you order an anti-Xa assay and it comes back at 0.82 units/mL.

a) What course of action will you take?

b) Include all calculations.

41) At 0400 the following day another anti-Xa assay is ordered and comes back at 0.75 units/mL.

a) Will you, or the on-duty nurse, adjust the dose?

b) If so, what will the new infusion rate be in units/h?

42) At 1000 another anti-Xa assay is ordered which comes back at 0.69 units/mL. What do you do?

Pt A.C., who weighs 107 kg, has been admitted with a diagnosis of DVT and has the following heparin order:
Initial bolus: 80 units/kg (max 10,000 units)
Initial infusion: 18 units/kg/h (initial max of 1800 units/h)

43) Calculate the bolus dose in units.

44) Calculate the bolus dose in mL.

45) Calculate the initial infusion rate in units/h.

46) Calculate the initial infusion rate in mL/h.

47) The initial infusion was started at 0915. At 1515 you order an anti-Xa assay and it comes back at 0.25 units/mL.

a) What is your course of action?

b) Include all calculations.

48) At 2115 another anti-Xa assay is ordered and comes back at 0.46 units/mL.

a) Will you, or the on-duty nurse, adjust the dose?

b) If so, what will the new infusion rate be in units/h?

49) At 0315 another anti-Xa assay is ordered which comes back at 0.44 units/mL. What do you do?

Pt W.W., who weighs 64 kg, has been admitted with a diagnosis of DVT and has the following heparin order:
Initial bolus: 80 units/kg (max 10,000 units)
Initial infusion: 18 units/kg/h (initial max of 1800 units/h)

50) Calculate the bolus dose in units.

51) Calculate the bolus dose in mL.

52) Calculate the initial infusion rate in units/h.

53) Calculate the initial infusion rate in mL/h.

54) The initial infusion was started at 0600. At 1200 you order an anti-Xa assay and it comes back at 0.84 units/mL.

a) What is your course of action?

b) What will the new infusion rate be in units/h?

55) At 1800 another anti-Xa assay is ordered and comes back at 0.74 units/mL.

a) Will you, or the on-duty nurse, adjust the dosage?

b) If so, what will the new infusion rate be in units/h?

56) At 0000 another anti-Xa assay is ordered which comes back at 0.72 units/mL.

a) Will you, or the on-duty nurse, adjust the dosage?

b) If so, what will the new infusion rate be in units/h?

Unit 6: Percent and Ratio Strength Calculations

Calculations involving percent are common in nursing calculations and seem to cause unnecessary anxiety. You won't learn to move the decimal point in this unit, but you will learn how to set up and solve the problems using mathematically correct equations.

Chapter 27: Percent
Summary: Explains the basics of percent and the power of multiplying and dividing by 100%.
Importance: 10/10.

Chapter 28: Percent Strength
Summary: Explains percent strength and how to set up and solve these problems.
Importance: 9/10

Chapter 29: Percent Change
Summary: Explains percent change and how to calculate it.
Importance: 9/10

Chapter 30: Ratio Strength
Summary: Explains ratio strength and the method to set up and solve these problems.
Importance: 10/10

Chapter 27
Percent

The three key concepts in understanding percent are:

- **Percent means per 100.** 50% is 50 parts per 100, or $\frac{50}{100}$.

- **100% equals 1.** Since 100% = 1, the corresponding conversion factors are $\left(\frac{100\%}{1}\right)$ and $\left(\frac{1}{100\%}\right)$, which is the same as multiplying or dividing by 100%.

- **The percent sign (%) will cancel itself out just as the units of measurement cancel themselves out.** $\frac{12\%}{100\%} = \frac{12}{100}$

Converting a Number to a Percent

- Convert a number to a percent by multiplying by 100%.
- Example: Convert 0.30 to a percent.   0.30 (100%) = 30%.
  - 100% = 1, so the value of 0.30 has not changed, only the appearance.

Converting a Percent to a Number

- Convert a percent to a number by dividing by 100%. If you wish, you can multiply by $\left(\frac{1}{100\%}\right)$, which is the same thing.
- Example: Convert 35% to a number.

$$\left(\frac{35\%}{100\%}\right) = 0.35.$$

Converting a Fraction to a Percent

- Convert a fraction to a percent by multiplying the fraction by 100%.
- Example: Convert 1/4 to a percent.   1/4 (100%) = 25%

Summing up: To add the % sign, multiply by 100%. To remove the % sign, divide by 100%. (Yes, you multiply or divide by 100%, NOT 100.)

Percent Exercise

Convert the following numbers to percents.

Problem	Number	Percent
Example	0.46	0.46 (100%) = 46%
1	0.42	
2	0.68	
3	1.392	
4	2.82	
5	0.005	
6	0.036	
7	1.29	
8	0.463	
9	0.549	
10	1.517	

Convert the following percents to numbers.

Problem	Percent	Number
Example	31%	31%/100% = 0.31
11	32.4%	
12	68%	
13	1.2%	
14	34.3%	
15	9.6%	
16	65.35%	
17	1.9%	
18	3.8%	
19	1.8%	
20	0.6%	

Chapter 28
Percent Strength

The only difference between percent strength and percent is that percent strength includes units of weight and volume.

- **Weight, in a percent strength, is always expressed in units of gram (g).**
- **Volume, in a percent strength, is always expressed in units of milliliter (mL).**

The Four Types of Mixtures, also Called Solutions

Weight in Weight $\left(\frac{w}{w}\right)$: An example is 1 g of hydrocortisone (the solute) in 100 g of final cream (the solution). This is a 1% hydrocortisone cream. When working with w/w calculations, it is best to label the weights with AI (for active ingredient) and the type of solution to distinguish the two. The 1% HC cream could be labeled 1 g AI/100 g cr.

Weight in Volume $\left(\frac{w}{v}\right)$: An example is 1 g of NaCl (the solute) in 100 mL of NaCl solution (the solution). This is a 1% NaCl solution.

Volume in Volume $\left(\frac{v}{v}\right)$: An example is 1 mL of ethanol (the solute) in 100 mL of final product (the solution) (1 mL ethanol mixed with 99 mL of water). This is a 1% ethanol solution.

Volume in weight $\left(\frac{v}{w}\right)$: This type of solution is not very common. An example is 10 mL of glycerin in 100 g glycerin ointment. This is a 10% glycerin ointment.

A 1% NaCl solution is 1% $\frac{w}{v}$ NaCl solution. Sometimes the units $\frac{w}{w}, \frac{w}{v}, \frac{v}{v}, \frac{v}{w}$ are not included in the problem and must be added. If it is weighed, it is w, if the volume is measured, it is v. Note that occasionally liquids are expressed in weight.

The Key to Solving these Problems

- **Substitute g for w and mL for v in the ratios and units of the answer.**
- **Preform the calculations.**
- **Substitute w and v back in the final answer, if required.**

Example: How many grams of NaCl are in 45 mL of $2\%\frac{w}{v}$ NaCl solution?

- This problem can be completed in one step. Substitute g for w and mL for v, multiply by 45 mL and divide by 100%.

$$45\,\text{mL} \left(\frac{2\%\ \text{g}}{100\%\ \text{mL}}\right) = 0.9\ \text{g}$$

See how nicely mL and % cancel out? If the problem asked for the number of mg, add the conversion factor $\left(\frac{1000\ \text{mg}}{\text{g}}\right)$.

$$45\,\text{mL} \left(\frac{2\%\ \text{g}}{100\%\ \text{mL}}\right)\left(\frac{1000\ \text{mg}}{\text{g}}\right) = 900\ \text{mg}$$

You will quickly realize that a 2% w/v solution is 2 g/100 mL, a 4% v/v solution is 4 mL Al/100 mL solution, etc., and it is easier to start with these ratios when doing the calculations.

Calculate the Percent Strength from Weight and Volume

Calculate the percent strength of a solution by setting up the problem with the given and the units of the answer. The final units of the answer will be % w/v, % w/w, % v/v, or % v/w, but substitute g and mL for w and v.

Example: What is the percent strength of a solution if there are 985 mg of NaCl in 2.5 L?

- Write down the given and the units of the answer:

$$\frac{985\ \text{mg}}{2.5\ \text{L}} = \%\ \frac{\text{g}}{\text{mL}}$$

It is now easy to see that mg must be converted to g, L converted to mL, and the % must be added.

- Convert mg to g by multiplying by $\left(\frac{1\ \text{g}}{1000\ \text{mg}}\right)$.
- Convert L to mL by multiplying by $\left(\frac{1\ \text{L}}{1000\ \text{mL}}\right)$.
- Add the % sign by multiplying by 100%.

$$\frac{985\,\text{mg}}{2.5\,\text{L}}\left(\frac{1\ \text{g}}{1000\,\text{mg}}\right)\left(\frac{1\,\text{L}}{1000\ \text{mL}}\right)100\% = 0.0394\%\ \frac{\text{g}}{\text{mL}}$$

- Substitute w for g and v for mL in the final answer: $0.0394\%\ \frac{w}{v}$

Percent Strength Exercise

Express the following as percent strength solutions and include the type of solution (w/w, w/v, v/v, v/w).

1) 1.5 g HC in 200 g HC ointment

2) 6.5 g NaCl in 1000 mL

3) 25 mL ETOH in 100 mL ETOH solution

4) 2.5 mg betamethasone in 5 g betamethasone ointment

5) 4.5 g NaCl in 2 L

6) 25 mcg NaCl in 0.25 mL

7) 500 mg NaHCO$_3$ in 200 mL

8) 5 g KCl in 200 mL

9) 10 g salicylic acid in 250 g salicylic acid cream

10) 10 g urea in 40 g urea ointment

Answer the following:

11) How many mg of lidocaine are in 300 mL of 1% lidocaine?

12) How many g of KCl are in 400 mL of 10% KCl?

13) How many mg of bupivacaine are in 60 mL of 0.5% bupivacaine solution?

14) How many g of HC are in 200 g of 2.5% HC ointment?

15) How many grams of dextrose are in 2.5 L of D5W (5% dextrose in water)?

16) How many mg of triamcinolone are in 45 g of 0.1% triamcinolone ointment?

17) How many mcg of dextrose are in 1 drop of 5% dextrose solution if there are 20 drops/mL?

18) How many g of NaCl are in 1.75 L of NS (normal saline-0.9% NaCl)?

19) How many mcg of fluocinolone are in 50 g of 0.01% fluocinolone cream?

20) How many mg of NaCl are in 50 mL of 0.9% NaCl (normal saline)?

Chapter 29
Percent Change

Occasionally you will be required to calculate the percent change between two quantities.

Example 1) A patient's weight increased from 81 kg to 84 kg. What is the percent change?

- The formula to calculate percent change is:

$$\frac{\text{Final} - \text{Initial}}{\text{Initial}} (100\%) = \% \text{ Change}$$

- The patient's final weight is 84 kg.
- The patient's initial weight is 81 kg.

$$\frac{84 \text{ kg} - 81 \text{ kg}}{81 \text{ kg}} (100\%) = \frac{3 \text{ kg}}{81 \text{ kg}} (100\%) = 3.7\%$$

Notice how if the units are the same, they cancel out? If the units are the same, which they usually are in these problems, it is ok to leave them out of the calculation. This is an exception to the rule in the introduction.

Example 2) A patient is prescribed 2.5 mg of a drug and the prescriber increased the dose to 3 mg. What is the percent change?

$$\frac{3 - 2.5}{2.5} (100\%) = \frac{0.5}{2.5} (100\%) = 20\%$$

Percent Change Exercise

Calculate the percent change in the following scenarios. Round to the nearest tenth percent.

1) You had to adjust an IV drip from 36 gtts/min to 40 gtts/min.

2) Your patient weighed 184 lb on admission and weighs 180 lb today.

3) A patient's daily dose of a drug was reduced from 50 mg to 40 mg.

4) A patient weighed 77 kg on Monday and still weighs 77 kg on Thursday.

5) You increase an IV flow rate from 10.5 mL/h to 13 mL/h.

6) The number of donuts in the breakroom decreased from 6 to 1 (the one nobody wants).

7) Your patient weighed 85 kg on admission and weighs 82 kg today.

8) You got a merit raise from $46.45/h to $48.05/h.

9) The number of patients in your unit increased from 8 to 12.

10) Your patient, who you encouraged to exercise and watch his diet, weighed 215 lb one month ago and now weighs 204 lb.

11) A dosage increased from 15 mg b.i.d to 20 mg b.i.d.

12) You start a diet and reduce your caloric intake from 4500 kcal/day to 2500 kcal/day.

13) You can now do 25 pushups but a month ago you could only do 15.

14) A patient had his atorvastatin dosage lowered from 80 mg once daily to 40 mg once daily.

15) You increased a Pitocin drip from 2 milliunits/minute to 3 milliunits/minute.

Chapter 30
Ratio Strength

- Occasionally, drug strengths are expressed as ratio strengths.
- These calculations have similarities to percent strength calculations.
    - The units are always g and mL.
    - Solutions may be w/w, w/v, v/v, or v/w.
- The conventional format is 1:another number, where the other number is the amount of final product. Examples: 1:100, 1:500, 1:10,000.
    - A 1:100 w/w preparation is 1 g active ingredient in 100 g of final product. **It is not 1 g of active ingredient mixed with 100 g of inactive ingredient.**
    - A 1:100 w/v solution is 1 g active ingredient in 100 mL solution.
    - A 1:100 v/v solution is 1 mL of active ingredient in 100 mL solution.
    - A 1:100 v/w solution is 1 mL of active ingredient in 100 g of product.
- **Keys to preforming calculations involving ratio strengths.**
    - Determine the type of solution (w/w, w/v, v/v, v/w).
    - Assign the units of g to w and mL to v.
    - Convert from the colon format into the fraction format with the units attached. **Example: 1:1000 w/v becomes 1 g/1000 mL.**
    - Proceed with calculations using DA or RP.

Example: How many mg of epinephrine are in 45 mL of a 1:10,000 solution of epinephrine?

- This is a **w** (mg) of epinephrine in **v** (45 mL) solution.
- 1:10,000 w/v is 1 g:10,000 mL
- 1 g:10,000 mL converted to fraction format is $\left(\frac{1\ g}{10,000\ mL}\right)$.
- Proceed with calculations using DA.

$$45\ mL \left(\frac{1\ g}{10,000\ mL}\right)\left(\frac{1000\ mg}{g}\right) = 4.5\ mg$$

Important: Many fatalities have resulted from incorrect calculations involving ratio strength, with epinephrine being one of the most common drugs involved. Be very careful when preforming ratio strength calculations. Most drugs labeled with ratio strength will include the strength listed in mg/mL, which is safer to use.

Ratio Strength Exercise

1) How many grams of active ingredient are in 350 g of a 1:50 w/w preparation?

2) You have a 100 mL vial which is labeled 1:1000. How many mg are in 60 mL of the solution?

3) How many mcg are in 120 mL of a 1:100,000 solution?

4) You have a 5 mL vial which is labeled 1:10,000 and are asked to draw up 0.4 mg of drug. How many mL would you draw?

5) How many mg of active ingredient are in 500 mL of a 1:10,000 solution?

6) How many grams of active ingredient are in 50 mL of a 1:200 solution?

7) How many grams of active ingredient are in 200 mL of a 1:10,000 solution?

8) You have a 50 mL vial which is labeled 1:1000 and are asked to draw up 1.4 mg. How many mL would you draw?

9) You have a solution which is 1:1000 w/v. What is the percent strength?

10) What is the percent strength of a 1:100 w/v solution?

Unit 7: Miscellaneous Subjects

These are the chapters which don't fit nicely into the previous units.

Chapter 31: Reconstitution Calculations
Summary: This is an easy chapter and was only added because these problems occur on nursing tests.
Importance: 8/10.

Chapter 32: Concentrations and Dilutions
Summary: This chapter covers concentrations and dilutions, probably in more detail than needed, but a basic understanding of this subject will come in handy.
Importance: 7/10

Chapter 33: Milliequivalent Calculations
Summary: This chapter explains milliequavlents (mEq) and how to convert between them and milligrams. You probably won't be asked to convert between mg and mEq on a test or in a clinical setting, but you should understand what a mEq is.
Importance: 6/10

Chapter 34: Dosage Calculation Puzzles
Summary: This chapter was added for those of you who have mastered everything else and want a challenge. Don't spend any time on these unless you understand everything else in the book.
Importance: 0/10

Chapter 35: Self-Assessment Exam
Summary: A self-assessment exam to highlight your strengths and weaknesses.
Importance: 9/10

Chapter 31
Reconstitution Calculations

Some drugs come in a dry form and must be reconstituted before administration. The instructions for reconstitution will either be supplied with the drug or available in a data base and must be followed exactly.

The basic method of solving these problems:

- Reconstitute the drug according to the instructions.
- Look at the final concentration and volume when doing the calculations. Forget about the amount of diluent you added in the first step as this has nothing to do with the dosage calculations.
- Note: If you are given a nursing student test question which only gives the amount of diluent, with no information on the final volume or concentration, you do not have enough information to solve the problem. You can't assume that the diluent volume is equal to the final volume.

Example: A 500 mg vial has directions to reconstitute with 1.8 mL of diluent for a final concentration of 250 mg/mL. You have an order for 300 mg. How many mL will you withdraw to administer this dose?

$$300 \text{ mg} \left(\frac{1 \text{ mL}}{250 \text{ mg}} \right) = 1.2 \text{ mL}$$

Once you have reconstituted the vial, the amount of diluent is not a factor in the dosage calculation.

Reconstitution Calculations Exercise

1) The physician has ordered 200 mg IM of a drug which is available in 1 g vials with instructions to add 3.6 mL SW for injection for a final concentration of 250 mg/mL. How many mL will you administer?

2) The physician has ordered 400 mg IM of a drug which is available in a 1000 mg vial with directions to add 4.3 mL SW for injection for a final concentration of 200 mg/mL. How many mL will you administer?

3) You have an order for 500 mg IV of a drug which is available in 1 g vials with directions to reconstitute with 8.5 mL of SW for injection for a final concentration of 100 mg/mL. How many mL will you administer?

4) A 1,000,000-unit vial of penicillin G potassium has instructions which state to reconstitute to a concentration of 100,000 units per mL, add 10 mL SW for injection. You have an order for 300,000 units IM. How many mL will you administer?

5) A 2 g vial states to add 7.4 mL of SW for injection for a final concentration of 200 mg/mL. You have an order for 250 mg IV. How many mL will you administer?

6) A 61 kg male patient diagnosed with herpes simplex encephalitis is to receive acyclovir 10 mg/kg IV infused over 1 hour, every 8 hours for 10 days. You have on hand a 1000 mg vial with the instructions to dissolve the contents of the vial in 20 mL of SWFI with the resulting solution containing 50 mg of acyclovir per mL. The calculated dose will then be withdrawn and added to a 100 mL bag of D5W. After reconstitution, what volume of the 50 mg/mL solution will you add to the 100 mL bag?

7) You are reconstituting a 150 mL bottle of amoxicillin 250 mg/5 mL. The instructions for reconstitution are as follows. Total amount of water required for reconstitution is 111 mL. Tap the bottle until all powder flows freely. Add approximately 1/3 of the total amount of water for reconstitution and shake vigorously to wet the powder. Add the remainder of the water and again shake vigorously. How many doses are contained in the bottle if the child were to take 6 mL PO t.i.d.?

8) A patient has an order for azithromycin 500 mg IV administered over 60 minutes at a concentration of 1 mg/mL. The 500 mg vial states: Prepare the initial solution of azithromycin for injection by adding 4.8 mL of Sterile Water For Injection to the vial and shaking the vial until all of the drug is dissolved. Each mL of the solution contains 100 mg of azithromycin.

a) The 5 mL vial will now be added to what size bag of NS to achieve a 1 mg/mL concentration?

b) At what rate will you set the IV infusion pump to the nearest tenth mL/h?

9) A patient has an order for streptomycin 500 mg IM which is available in 1 g vials with instructions to add 3.2 mL of Water for Injection USP for a final concentration of 250 mg/mL. How many mL will you administer?

10) You have an order for 350 mg IM of a drug which is available in a 500 mg vial with instructions to add 4.4 mL of SW for injection for a final concentration of 100 mg/mL. How many mL will you administer?

Chapter 32
Concentrations and Dilutions

This chapter covers calculations involving concentrations, dilution, and mixing. There are several different types of problems in this chapter, but they all have similar components.

Topics covered are:

- **The Alligation Method**
  - A method used to calculate the volumes of two different strength solutions when preparing a third strength. It may also be used on some simpler problems.
- **Preparing a Solution Using Two Different Strength Solutions**
  - This topic is covered in the alligation method.
- **Preparing a Solution Using a Stock Solution and a Diluent**
  - This is the most common type of dilution calculation encountered. Several different methods of solving these problems will be explained.
- **Calculating the Percent Strength of a Mixture**
  - These calculations seem complicated at first but are very easy.

The Alligation Method

- **The alligation method is an easy way of solving problems which involve mixing two different strength solutions to form a third strength.**
- **Although not usually the easiest method of solving simple dilution problems, it can be used for these problems if desired.**
- **All strengths must be in percent strength.**

Example: How much 10% solution must be mixed with a 25% solution to prepare 1000 mL of a 22% solution

Step 1) Draw a box and place the percent of the lower strength solution on the lower left corner, the percent of the higher strength solution on the upper left corner, and the percent of the of the solution being preparing in the middle. In the above example, a 10 is placed in the lower left corner, a 25 in the upper left corner and a 22 in the middle.

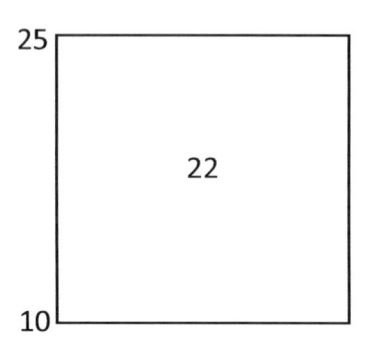

```
25 ┌─────────┐
   │         │
   │    22   │
   │         │
10 └─────────┘
```

Step 2) Take the difference between the lower left corner and the middle and write it in the upper right corner. Take the difference between the upper left corner and the middle and write it in the lower right corner. Note: The differences are always written as positive numbers.

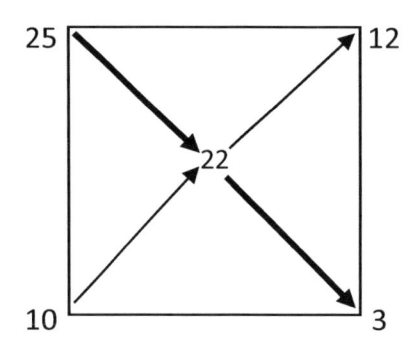

```
25 ┌─────────┐ 12
   │    22   │
10 └─────────┘ 3
```

Step 3) The 12 and the 3 represent the number of parts of the 25% solution and the 10% solution needed to make the 22% solution. The total number of parts of both solutions is 15 (12 + 3), so 12/15 of the final solution is the 25% solution and 3/15 of the final solution is the 10% solution. Multiply 1000 mL by 12/15 to determine the amount of 25% solution. Multiply 1000 mL by 3/15 to determine the amount of 10% solution to add.

$$1000 \text{ mL} \left(\frac{12}{15}\right) = 800 \text{ mL of } 25\% \text{ solution}$$

$$1000 \text{ mL} \left(\frac{3}{15}\right) = 200 \text{ mL of } 10\% \text{ solution}$$

This method can also be used when preparing a solution from a stock solution and a diluent if the stock solution and final product are expressed in percent strength. Use a 0 in the lower left corner and the percent strength of the stock solution in the upper left corner.

Preparing a Solution from a Stock Solution and a Diluent

This is probably the most common type of dilution problem encountered. Three common methods of solving these problems are:

- Calculate amount of active ingredient in the final product, then calculate amount of stock solution required to obtain the active ingredient.
- Use the formula V1C1=V2C2, where V1=volume of first solution, C1=concentration of first solution, V2=volume of second solution, C2=concentration of second solution.
- Use the alligation method, which is not the easiest or quickest way.

Consider the following example solved using each of the three methods.

An order calls for 600 mL of a 25 mg/mL solution. You have a 100 mg/mL stock solution on hand. How many mL of the stock solution and how many mL of the diluent are needed?

Method 1: Calculate the amount of active ingredient in the final product then calculate the volume of stock solution needed to obtain that amount of active ingredient.

$$600 \text{ mL} \left(\frac{25 \text{ mg}}{\text{mL}}\right) = 15,000 \text{ mg}$$

15,000 mg of active ingredient is in the final product. The volume of stock solution required to obtain the 15,000 mg of active ingredient is now calculated.

$$15,000 \text{ mg} \left(\frac{1 \text{ mL}}{100 \text{ mg}}\right) = 150 \text{ mL}$$

150 mL of the stock solution will be mixed with 450 mL (600 mL – 150 mL) of diluent to prepare the final solution.

Method 2: Use the formula V1C1=V2C2. In this case, V1=600 mL, C1=25 mg/mL, V2 is unknown stock solution volume and C2 is 100 mg/mL.

$$600 \text{ mL} \left(\frac{25 \text{ mg}}{\text{mL}}\right) = V2 \left(\frac{100 \text{ mg}}{\text{mL}}\right)$$

To solve for V2, multiply both sides by 1 mL/100 mL.

$$V2 = 600 \text{ mL} \left(\frac{25 \text{ mg}}{\text{mL}}\right)\left(\frac{1 \text{ mL}}{100 \text{ mg}}\right)$$

V2=150 mL

This method works because VC=AI (Active Ingredient). The AI is the same in both solutions.

Method 3: Convert the stock solution and the final solution concentrations to percent strength, then use the alligation method.

The stock solution is 100 mg/mL.

$$\frac{100 \text{ mg}}{\text{mL}} \left(\frac{1 \text{ g}}{1000 \text{ mg}}\right) 100\% = 10\% \frac{\text{g}}{\text{mL}} = 10\% \frac{\text{w}}{\text{v}}$$

The final preparation is 25 mg/mL, which works out to 2.5% w/v.

The diluent is 0%.

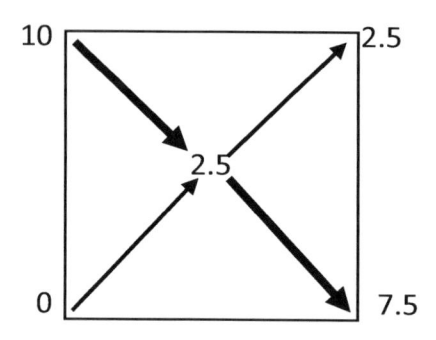

```
10 ─────────── 2.5
   ╲         ╱
    ╲       ╱
     ╲ 2.5 ╱
     ╱     ╲
    ╱       ╲
   ╱         ╲
 0 ─────────── 7.5
```

The total parts are 10, with 2.5/10 being the 10% solution and 7.5/10 being the 0% (diluent).

$$600 \text{ mL} \left(\frac{2.5}{10}\right) = 150 \text{ mL of } 10\% \text{ solution}$$

$$600 \text{ mL} \left(\frac{7.5}{10}\right) = 450 \text{ mL of } 0\% \text{ solution}$$

- If all the solutions are stated in percent strength, you might consider using this method, otherwise it is easier to use one of the first two methods.

Calculating the Percent Strength of a Mixture

To calculate the final concentration of a mixture of two or more solutions with different strengths, the amount of active ingredient and the volume of the final solution must be determined.

Example: 100 mL of a 40% w/v solution, 25 mL of a 90% w/v solution and 40 mL of a 75% w/v solution are mixed together. What is the percent strength of the final solution?

- Start by calculating the amount of active ingredient in each of the three solutions.

$$100 \text{ mL} \left(\frac{40 \text{ g}}{100 \text{ mL}}\right) = 40 \text{ g}$$

$$25 \text{ mL} \left(\frac{90 \text{ g}}{100 \text{ mL}}\right) = 22.5 \text{ g}$$

$$40 \text{ mL} \left(\frac{75 \text{ g}}{100 \text{ mL}}\right) = 30 \text{ g}$$

- Total the volumes and active ingredients of the three solutions.
  - 100 mL + 25 mL + 40 mL = 165 mL
  - 40 g + 22.5 g + 30 g = 92.5 g
- Convert 92.5 g/165 mL into a percent strength.

$$\frac{92.5 \text{ g}}{165 \text{ mL}} (100\%) = 56.1\% \frac{\text{g}}{\text{mL}} = 56.1\% \frac{\text{w}}{\text{v}}$$

Concentration and Dilution Exercise

1) An order calls for 600 mL of a 15% solution. You have a 40% solution on hand. How many mL of stock solution (40%) and how many mL of diluent are needed?

2) You have on hand a 35% stock solution. A doctor writes an order for 60 mL of a 25% solution. How many mL of the stock solution and how many mL of diluent are needed?

3) An order is written for 300 mL of a 7.5% solution. You have a 50% solution available. How many mL of the stock solution and how many mL of diluent are needed?

4) You have an order for 100 mL of a 50 mg/mL solution. Your stock bottle is labeled 300 mg/2 mL. How many mL of the stock solution and how many mL of diluent are needed?

5) The provider has ordered 3/4 strength tube-feeding formula for your patient. You have available a 240 mL container. How much water will you add to the 240 mL to prepare the 3/4 strength formula?

6) The pharmacy stocks a 15% and a 75% solution. You receive an order for 300 mL of a 35% solution, but the pharmacy is too busy to help you. How many milliliters of the 15% and 75% solutions are needed?

7) An order is written for 500 mL of a 34% solution. Your pharmacy stocks a 10% and a 45% solution. How many milliliters of the 10% and 45% solutions are needed?

8) What is the percentage strength of a mixture containing 80 mL of a 10% solution and 180 mL of a 35% solution?

9) The provider has ordered 1/2 strength tube-feeding formula for your patient. You have available a 240 mL container. How much water will you add to the 240 mL to prepare the 1/2 strength formula?

10) What is the percent strength of a mixture containing 100 mL of a 7% solution, 200 mL of a 10% solution and 700 mL of a 15% solution, all the same active ingredient?

Chapter 33
Milliequivalent Calculations

As nurses, you will probably not be required to convert between mg and mEq, but some of you may want to go above and beyond what is required. If nothing else, learning the terminology and key concepts listed below will be helpful.

Terminology:

- **Electrolytes:** Ions which are important to the function of the body. (Na^+, K^+, Cl^-, etc.)
- **Ion:** An atom or group of atoms that has either lost or gained electrons and carries either a positive or negative charge.
- **Cation:** A positively charged ion (pronounced cat-ion).
- **Anion:** A negatively charged ion.
- **Valence:** The simple definition is the number of charges on the ion.
- **Atomic Mass/Atomic Weight:** For purposes of this book, these terms are used interchangeably. They are relative weights of the elements. For example, hydrogen has an atomic mass of 1 while carbon has an atomic mass of 12. An atom of carbon is twelve times as heavy as an atom of hydrogen. There are no units on atomic masses.

Key Concepts to Understanding Milliequivalent Calculations

- mEq calculations involve quantities of ions and charges, not weights. Think dozens of eggs, not pounds of coffee beans.
- A millimole (mmole) is 1/1000 of a mole (mol) or 6.022×10^{20} of anything.
- A mEq is a mmol of charges.
  Examples:
- 1 mmol of NaCl = 1 mmol of Na^+ and 1 mmol of Cl^-.
- Na^+ and Cl^- each have one charge.
- 1 mmol of NaCl = 1 mEq of Na^+ and 1 mEq Cl^-.
- 1 mmol of $MgSO_4$ = 1 mmol of Mg^{+2} and 1 mmol of SO_4^{-2}.
- Mg^{+2} and SO_4^{-2} each have two charges.
- 1 mmol of $MgSO_4$ = 2 mEq of Mg^{+2} and 2 mEq of SO_4^{-2}.

Converting Between mg and mEq

- The weight of a mmol of the electrolyte and the valence must be known.
- Determine the weight of a mmol of the electrolyte by looking up the atomic mass and adding mg to the end to give you the mg/mmol. For example, the atomic mass of potassium (K) is 39.1, which equates to 39.1 mg/mmol.
- Determine the valence by looking it up. The common electrolytes and their valences are listed in the milliequivalent exercise.

Example: How many mEq of KCl are in 300 mg of KCl?

- The formula mass (mass of $K^+ + Cl^-$) is 74.6, meaning 74.6 mg = 1 mmol. There is one charge on each ion, so 1 mmol = 1 mEq.

$$300 \text{ mg}\left(\frac{1 \text{ mmol}}{74.6 \text{ mg}}\right)\left(\frac{1 \text{ mEq}}{\text{mmol}}\right) = 4 \text{ mEq}$$

- It can also be stated that 4 mEq of KCl = 4 mEq of K^+ and 4 mEq of Cl^-.

Example: How many mEq of Mg^{+2} are in 300 mg of $MgSO_4$?

$$300 \text{ mg}\left(\frac{1 \text{ mmol}}{120.4 \text{ mg}}\right)\left(\frac{2 \text{ mEq}}{\text{mmol}}\right) = 5 \text{ mEq}$$

Milliequivalent Calculations Exercise

1) Look up the atomic masses (atomic weights) of the following elements. The atomic masses can be found on the periodic table or Google it. If you can't find them on your own, they are listed in the answers. Round to the nearest tenth.

Name	Atomic Symbol	Atomic Mass	Ionic Form
Hydrogen	H		H^+ (Hydrogen Ion)
Carbon	C		
Oxygen	O		
Sodium	Na		Na^+ (Sodium Ion)
Magnesium	Mg		Mg^{++} (Magnesium Ion)
Chlorine	Cl		Cl^- (Chloride Ion)
Potassium	K		K^+ (Potassium Ion)
Calcium	Ca		Ca^{++} (Calcium Ion)
Sulfur	S		

2) Now that you know the atomic masses of each of the elements, fill in the formula masses of the listed polyatomic ions (ions with more than one atom). Add up all the individual masses. CH_3COO^- has two carbon atoms, three hydrogen atoms, and two oxygen atoms.

Name	Chemical Formula	Formula Mass	Ionic Form
Acetate	CH_3COO^-		CH_3COO^-
Bicarbonate	HCO_3^-		HCO_3^-
Sulfate	SO_4^{-2}		SO_4^{-2}

3) Now that you know the above atomic and formula masses, you are ready to list the formula masses of the following ionic compounds.

Name	Chemical Formula	Formula Mass	Ionic Form
Sodium Chloride	NaCl		$Na^+ Cl^-$
Potassium Chloride	KCl		$K^+ Cl^-$
Calcium Chloride	$CaCl_2$		$Ca^{++} 2Cl^-$
Magnesium Chloride	$MgCl_2$		$Mg^{++} 2Cl^-$
Sodium Acetate	CH_3COONa		$Na^+ CH_3COO^-$
Potassium Acetate	CH_3COOK		$K^+ CH_3COO^-$
Magnesium Sulfate	$MgSO_4$		$Mg^{++} SO_4^{2-}$
Sodium Bicarbonate	$NaHCO_3$		$Na^+ HCO_3^-$

4) Fill in the table with the ratios of mg/mmol and mEq/mmol for each compound.

Name	Chemical Formula	mg/mmol (ratio)	mEq/mmol (ratio)
Sodium Chloride	NaCl		
Potassium Chloride	KCl		
Calcium Chloride	$CaCl_2$		
Magnesium Chloride	$MgCl_2$		
Sodium Acetate	CH_3COONa		
Potassium Acetate	CH_3COOK		
Magnesium Sulfate	$MgSO_4$		
Sodium Bicarbonate	$NaHCO_3$		

- You now have all the ratios needed to convert between mg and mEq.

Example: How many mEq are in 500 mg of CaCl₂?

- Calcium chloride has 111 mg per mmol and two mEq per mmol.
- These ratios can be written $\frac{111 \text{ mg}}{\text{mmol}}$ or $\frac{1 \text{ mmol}}{111 \text{ mg}}$ and $\frac{2 \text{ mEq}}{\text{mmol}}$ or $\frac{1 \text{ mol}}{2 \text{ mEq}}$.
- Set the problem up with the given and units of the answer.

          500 mg   = mEq

- Insert the ratios in the usual way leaving only the units of the answer.

$$500 \text{ mg} \left(\frac{1 \text{ mmol}}{111 \text{ mg}}\right)\left(\frac{2 \text{ mEq}}{\text{mmol}}\right) = 9.0 \text{ mEq}$$

5) How many mEq of MgSO₄ are contained in 13 g of MgSO₄?

6) How many mEq of NaCl are in 2 L of 0.45% NaCl?

7) How many mEq of calcium chloride are contained in 2.5 g of calcium chloride?

8) How many mEq of Ca⁺⁺ are in 1.4 g of calcium chloride?

9) How many mEq of K⁺ are contained in 250 mg of KCl?

10) How many grams of Na⁺ (just the sodium) are contained in 3.5 L of 10% NaCl?

11) How many mg of magnesium sulfate are in 40 mEq of magnesium sulfate?

12) How many mEq of KCl are in 20 mL of 10% KCl solution?

13) How many g of sodium acetate are in 25 mEq of sodium acetate?

14) How many mg of KCl are in 60 mL of 2 mEq/mL KCl?

Chapter 34
Dosage Calculation Puzzles

These problems are just for fun and would never happen in a clinical setting.

1) You have an order to start an IV infusion at x mL/h, where 3x + 25= 175, on your patient Mr. Whipple, who is recovering from wrist surgery. The IV bag contains y mg/ z mL, where 3y + z = 620 and y-z = -460. Mr. Whipple weighs 73 kg. How many mcg/kg/min is Mr. receiving?

2) You have an order for 1 g of a drug to infuse over 4 hours. The pharmacy sends you a 1 L bag labeled: contains 250 mL of 3 mg/mL, 250 mL of 2 mg/mL, 250 mL of 5 mg/mL and 250 mL of NS.

a) At what rate will you set the pump?

b) You started the infusion at 1300. You check on the patient at 1400 only to learn that the patient turned off the pump at 1345 because his friend told him that he didn't need any big pharma drugs. After explaining the importance of the drug to the patient, you get out your calculator and note pad. At what rate will you set the pump to finish the 1 g infusion on time if you restart the infusion at 1415?

3) A new miracle drug is released by the FDA which reverses aging by 25% in adults over 50 YO. The dosage is 3 mg/kg + 2.5 mg for each year over 50 years old, rounded to the nearest 10 mg, given IV over 2 hours. The drug is available in 25 mg vials with instructions to reconstitute each vial with 8 mL of supplied diluent to yield a concentration of 2.5 mg/mL. Your facility's protocol is to reconstitute the appropriate number of vials and add to a 500 mL bag of D5W after withdrawing an equal volume of reconstituted drug from the 500 mL bag, then infuse over 2 hours. The drug, Youngme, is very expensive at $250/mg. Your facility has a new policy stating that the nurse who administers the drug must also calculate the charge of the drug and collect the cash payment. Your patient, Mr. Wrinkles, is 74 years old and weighs 80 kg. He is a little concerned about the price of the drug and relays to you that he makes $23.50/hour as a professional dog food taster. Mr. Wrinkles works 8 hours/day, five days per week. What will be the total charge for Mr. Wrinkles' therapy and how many weeks, days and hours will he have to work to pay for it?

Chapter 35
Self-Assessment Exam

The exam has 100 questions, each worth one point.

Convert the following:

1) 60 mL = L

2) 4.5 g = mg

3) 2 tbs = mL

4) 1.5 cups = mL

5) 120 mL = fl oz

6) 178 lb = kg

7) 8.5 cm = in

8) 1.85 kg = lb

9) 140 g = kg

10) 3 tbs = mL

Round the following numbers to the nearest tenth.

11) 6.43

12) 0.186

13) 5.96

14) 0.0005

15) 38.044

Round the following numbers to the nearest hundredth.

16) 16.874

17) 4.047

18) 31.006

19) 0.0565

20) 4.168

Write the corresponding Roman numerals for the following numbers:

21) 9

22) 4

23) 22

24) 43

25) 125

Write the corresponding numbers for the following Roman numerals:

26) VIII

27) LIX

28) XXXII

29) CXI

30) CX

Convert the following to scientific notation:

31) 320,000

32) 162,000,000

33) 0.0000054

34) 45,000

35) 249,000

Convert the following from scientific notation to numbers.

36) 8.34×10^5

37) 9.202×10^5

38) 2.302×10^{-6}

39) 5.15×10^{-8}

40) 6.104×10^7

Answer the following questions concerning military time.

41) You started studying for your exam at 1700 and finished at 2230. How many hours and minutes did you study?

42) What is 4:25 PM in military time?

43) You start and IV at 0800 which is scheduled to run 8 hours. What time will it end in military time?

44) A patient is to receive a medication every 8 hours around the clock. He received doses at 0600 and 1400. When should he receive the next dose?

45) You are asked to work from 10:00 AM to 1800. Your employer tells you that you can either be paid $37.50 per hour or a flat rate of $325. Which is the better deal for you?

Convert the following numbers to percents.

46) 0.06

47) 1.35

48) 0.475

Convert the following percents to numbers.

49) 83.1%

50) 100%

51) 0.152%

Express the following as percent strength solutions and include the type of solution (w/w, w/v, v/v, v/w).

52) 7.5 g NaCl in 1000 mL

53) 1.6 g KCl in 100 mL

54) 40 mL ETOH in 160 mL.

Answer the following:

55) How many mg of lidocaine are in 250 mL of 1% lidocaine solution?

56) How many mg of triamcinolone are in 45 g of 0.5% triamcinolone cream?

57) How many mg of NaCl are in 400 mL of 0.9% NaCl?

Answer the following questions pertaining to percent change.

58) You weigh 162 lb on August 1st and spend the next week hiking around Yosemite National Park. On August 8th you weigh 152 lb. What is the percent change in your weight?

59) You have two hamsters who fall in love and have 4 babies. What is the percent change in your hamster population?

60) The physician changed a patient's dose of a drug from 50 mg to 25 mg. What is the percent change in the dose?

61) Kristina F, a nursing student, scored 80% on her dosage calculation quiz on Monday. The following Monday she scored 98%. What is the percent change in her grade?

62) Your patient weighed 75 kg on admission and now weighs 73 kg. What is the percent change in the patient's weight?

Answer the following dosage questions.

63) The PCP has ordered 80 mg IM of a drug which is available in 200 mg/mL. How many mL will you administer?

64) The physician has ordered 40 mg IV of a drug which is available in 5 mL vials of 10 mg/mL. How many mL will you administer?

65) The NP ordered 80 mg PO once daily for a patient. The drug is available in 40 mg tablets. How many tablets will the patient take each day?

66) The physician has ordered 90 mg IM of a drug which is available in 10 mL vials containing 45 mg/mL. How many mL will you administer?

67) Your patient has an order for 12.5 mg PO of a drug which is available in 5 mg scored tablets. How many tabs will you administer?

68) Your 52 YO patient, who weighs 165 lb, has an order for drug xyz 100 mg/day divided into two doses. Drug xyz is available in 10 mL vials containing 40 mg/mL. How many mL will you administer per dose?

69) You have an order to administer 100 mcg/day PO divided into two doses. You have 0.025 mg tablets available. How many tablets will you administer per dose?

70) Your patient has an order for 250 mg IV every 6 hours of a drug which is available in 10 mL vials containing 25 mg/mL. How many mL will be administered in 24 hours?

71) The physician has ordered 500 mcg IM of a drug which is available in 2 mL vials containing 0.5 mg/mL. How many mL will you administer?

72) The physician has ordered 60 mg IV of a drug which is available in 5 mL vials containing 20 mg/mL. How many mL will you administer?

73) A 39 lb child has an order for furosemide 2 mg/kg PO once daily. Furosemide oral solution is available in 60 mL bottles containing 10 mg/mL. How many mL will you administer per dose?

74) A 78 kg patient is to receive an initial bolus dose of a drug 0.085 mg/kg over at least 2 minutes. The drug is available in 4 mL vials containing 2.5 mg/mL. How many mL will you administer?

75) A 155 lb patient is to receive a single IV dose of ondansetron 0.15 mg/kg for prevention of nausea and vomiting. Ondansetron is available in 20 mL MDV of 2 mg/mL. How many mL will you administer?

Calculate the flow rate in mL per hour rounded to the nearest tenth mL/h.

76) 1000 mL infused over 8 hours.

77) 500 mL infused over 7 hours.

78) 1000 mL infused over 6 hours.

79) 100 mL infused over 30 minutes.

Calculate the flow rate in drops/min. Round to the nearest whole drop.

80) 500 mL infused over 6 hours with a drop factor of 20 (20 gtts/mL).

81) 1000 mL infused over 5 hours with a drop factor of 10.

82) 250 mL infused over 3 hours with a drop factor of 15.

83) 500 mL infused over 8 hours with a microdrip set (60 gtts/mL).

Calculate the length of time in hours and minutes, rounded to the nearest minute, required to infuse the following:

84) 500 mL at 45 mL/h.

85) 750 mL at 90 mL/h.

86) 500 mL at 55 gtts/min with a drop factor of 20.

87) 1 L at 36 gtts/min with a drop factor of 15.

Calculate the volume infused in the following scenarios.

88) Infusion rate of 30 mL/h for 5 h 30 min.

89) Infusion rate of 28 gtts/min, drop factor 20, for 3 hours 45 min.

Calculate the following. Round all drops/min to the nearest drop and all mL/h rates to the nearest tenth mL/h.

90) Your 61 kg patient has an order for a lidocaine infusion at the rate of 20 mcg/kg/min. You have a 250 mL bag labeled "Lidocaine HCl and 5% Dextrose Injection USP". Lidocaine 2 g (8 mg/mL) is printed in big red letters in the middle of the label. What rate will you set the IV infusion pump?

91) Your 160 lb patient, who has been diagnosed with septic shock, has an order for norepinephrine 0.15 mcg/kg/min IV. The pharmacy delivers a bag containing 4 mg norepinephrine in 250 mL D5NS. At what rate will you set the IV infusion pump?

92) Your 172 lb female patient has an order for dobutamine 5 mcg/kg/min IV to start at 1300. The dobutamine is available as 1000 mcg/mL. At what rate will you set the IV infusion pump?

Answer the following reconstitution calculation questions.

93) You have an order for 150 mg IM of a drug which is available in 1 g vials with directions to reconstitute with 8.5 mL of SW for injection for a final concentration of 100 mg/mL. How many mL will you administer?

94) A patient has an order for 500 mg IM of a drug which is available in 1 g vials with instructions to add 3.2 mL of Water for Injection USP for a final concentration of 250 mg/mL. How many mL will you administer?

Calculate the BSA in m² for the following people using the Mosteller formula.

95) An adult male weighing 175 lb and 5 ft 11 in tall.

96) A 14-month-old girl weighing 22 lb and 30 in tall.

97) An adult male weighing 93 kg and 185 cm tall.

Answer the following:

98) The provider ordered 3/4 strength formula tube feeding for your patient. How much water would you add to a 180 mL container of full-strength formula?

99) A mEq of Na⁺ and a mEq of K⁺ weigh the same. T or F

100) A mEq of Na⁺ and a mEq of K⁺ contain the same number of ions. T or F

A Final Note

It is our hope that you found this book valuable and worthy of your study time. If so, please leave a review at www.nursesuperhero.com/dc2review. If not, please let us know how we can improve the book by contacting us at support@nursesuperhero.com.

Chase Hassen and Brad Wojcik

List of Abbreviations and Symbols

Term	Meaning	Term	Meaning
%	percent	mcg	microgram
AI	active ingredient	MD	Doctor of Medicine
AOM	acute otitis media	MDV	multiple dose vial
b.i.d.	twice daily	mg	milligram
BEACOPP	a chemotherapy regimen	mL	milliliter
BSA	body surface area	mm	millimeter
cap	capsule	NP	Nurse Practitioner
cm	centimeter	NPO	nothing orally
D5NS	5% dextrose in normal saline	NS	normal saline
D5W	5% dextrose in water	NTG	nitroglycerin
DCFMS	*Dosage Calculations for Nursing Students*	OM	otitis media
dL	deciliter	oz	ounce
DVT	deep vein thrombosis	p.	page
ETOH	ethyl alcohol	PA	Physician Assistant
fl oz	fluid ounce	PCI	percutaneous coronary intervention
g	gram	PE	pulmonary embolism
gal	gallon	PO	orally
gr	grain	pp.	pages
gtt	drop	pt	pint or patient
gtts	drops	q	every
G-tube	gastrostomy tube	q 2 h	every 2 hours
h	hour	q 6 h	every 6 hours
HC	hydrocortisone	q.i.d.	four times daily
HSE	herpes simplex encephalitis	STEMI	ST-Elevation Myocardial Infarction
IM	Intramuscularly	SW	sterile water
in	inch	SWFI	sterile water for injection
INR	international normalized ratio	t.i.d.	three times daily
IV	intravenously	tab	tablet
IVP	IV push	tbs	tablespoonful
kg	kilogram	tsp	teaspoonful
L	liter	VZV	varicella zoster virus
lb	pound	Xa	activated Factor X (ten)
LDL	low-density lipoprotein	YO	years old
m	meter		

Answers to Exercises
Chapter 5
Rounding Exercise

Problem	Round to the Nearest Tenth	Rounded Number	Problem	Round to the Nearest Hundredth	Rounded Number
Example	3.054	3.1	Example	78.386	78.39
1	121.16	**121.2**	26	8.875	**8.88**
2	4.37	**4.4**	27	3.295	**3.30**
3	10.26	**10.3**	28	5.111	**5.11**
4	89.43	**89.4**	28	35.589	**35.59**
5	6.57	**6.6**	30	9.598	**9.60**
6	87.449	**87.4**	31	0.297	**0.30**
7	0.3256	**0.3**	32	6.205	**6.21**
8	2.98	**3.0**	33	6.393	**6.39**
9	708.32	**708.3**	34	58.451	**58.45**
10	29.99	**30.0**	35	2.782	**2.78**
11	5.06	**5.1**	36	5.433	**5.43**
12	23.598	**23.6**	37	4.554	**4.55**
13	78.53	**78.5**	38	2.256	**2.26**
14	5.44	**5.4**	39	1.874	**1.87**
15	78.3	**78.3**	40	3.987	**3.99**
16	10.01	**10.0**	41	9.672	**9.67**
17	53.247	**53.2**	42	3.3595	**3.36**
18	0.88	**0.9**	43	1.005	**1.01**
19	2.22	**2.2**	44	4.956	**4.96**
20	9.355	**9.4**	45	1.8954	**1.90**
21	9.11	**9.1**	46	89.548	**89.55**
22	9.78	**9.8**	47	0.987	**0.99**
23	78.59	**78.6**	48	6.523	**6.52**
24	76.203	**76.2**	49	2.212	**2.21**
25	22.56	**22.6**	50	4.228	**4.23**

Dosage Calculations for Nursing Students-Second Edition

Chapter 6
Military Time Exercise

Convert the following civilian times to military time.

1) 3:15 AM   **0315**

2) 9:25 PM   **2125**

3) 8:13 AM   **0813**

4) 10:23 PM   **2223**

5) 4:49 AM   **0449**

Convert the following military times to civilian times.

6) 0422   **4:22 AM**

7) 2215   **10:15 PM**

8) 0905   **9:05 AM**

9) 0710   **7:10 AM**

10) 1310   **1:10 PM**

11) You started work at 0700 and you ended work at 1630. You didn't get any lunch or breaks (poor you). How many hours did you work?

9.5 hours

12) An IV was started at 1100 and ended at 3:30 PM. How many hours did it run?

4.5 hours

13) You have the weekend off. You started watching your favorite Netflix series at 0830 on Saturday morning and finished at 0030 on Sunday. How many hours did you sit on the couch watching TV?

16 hours

14) A patient is admitted at 0600 Monday morning and is discharged at 0800 the following morning. How many hours did the patient spend in the hospital?

26 hours

Chapter 7
Roman Numeral Exercise

1) You must know the eight basic Roman numerals and their number counterparts: SS, I, V, X, L, C, D, M.
Fill in the blanks in the following table.

Roman Numeral	Number	Number	Roman Numeral
SS	1/2	1/2 (0.5)	SS
I	1	1	I
V	5	5	V
X	10	10	X
L	50	50	L
C	100	100	C
D	500	500	D
M	1000	1000	M

2) Fill in the blanks with the corresponding Roman numerals or numbers.

50	L	C	100
100	C	5	V
1/2	SS	10	X
X	10	L	50
M	1000	I	1
5	V	X	10
V	5	D	500
500	D	M	1000
L	50	X	10
SS	½	V	5
1000	M	L	50
1	I	C	100
D	500	5	V
L	50	50	L
M	1000	1000	M
10	X	100	C

3) Fill in the blanks with the corresponding Roman numerals.

1000	M	100	C	10	X	1	I
2000	MM	200	CC	20	XX	2	II
3000	MMM	300	CCC	30	XXX	3	III
		400	CD	40	XL	4	IV
		500	D	50	L	5	V
		600	DC	60	LX	6	VI
		700	DCC	70	LXX	7	VII
		800	DCCC	80	LXXX	8	VIII
		900	CM	90	XC	9	IX
						1/2	SS

Dosage Calculations for Nursing Students-Second Edition

4) Fill in the blanks with the corresponding number or Roman numeral.

10	**X**	LXX	**70**
30	**XXX**	20	**XX**
400	**CD**	CCC	**300**
DC	**600**	CD	**400**
2000	**MM**	CM	**900**
8	**VIII**	700	**DCC**
XC	**90**	50	**L**
40	**XL**	20	**XX**
60	**LX**	LXXX	**80**
200	**CC**	DCC	**700**
900	**CM**	600	**DC**
IV	**4**	CC	**200**
III	**3**	9	**IX**
SS	**1/2**	4	**IV**

5) Write 1742 as a Roman numeral.

1000	M
700	DCC
40	XL
2	II

Answer: MDCCXLII

6) Write 2117 as a Roman numeral.

2000	MM
100	C
10	X
7	VII

Answer: MMCXVII

7) Write 2019 as a Roman numeral.

2000	MM
0	
10	X
9	IX

Answer: MMXIX

8) Write MDCCLXXVI as a number.

M	1000
DCC	700
LXX	70
VI	6

Answer: 1776

9) Write MCDXCII as a number.

M	1000
CD	400
XC	90
II	2

Answer: 1492

10) Write MCCXV as a number.

M	1000
CC	200
X	10
V	5

Answer: 1215

Chapter 8
Scientific Notation Exercise

1) Convert the following numbers to scientific notation.

Number	Coefficient	# of Places from New Decimal Point to end of Original Number	Coefficient X 10 Raised to the Number of Places the Decimal Point was Moved
67,000	6.7	4	6.7×10^4
8,247,000	8.247	6	8.247×10^6
1,150,000	1.15	6	1.15×10^6
94,800	9.48	4	9.48×10^4
732,000	7.32	5	7.32×10^5
921,000	9.21	5	9.21×10^5
38,300,000	3.83	7	3.83×10^7
2,470,000	2.47	6	2.47×10^6
92,500,000	9.25	7	9.25×10^7
49,230,000,000	4.923	10	4.923×10^{10}
125,000	1.25	5	1.25×10^5

2) Convert the following decimal numbers to scientific notation.

Decimal Number	Coefficient	# of Places from New Decimal Point to Original Decimal Point	Coefficient X 10 Raised to the Negative Number of Places the Decimal Point was Moved
0.056	5.6	2	5.6×10^{-2}
0.00580	5.80	3	5.80×10^{-3}
0.00070	7.0	4	7.0×10^{-4}
0.0004039	4.039	4	4.039×10^{-4}
0.005068	5.068	3	5.068×10^{-3}
0.0001332	1.332	4	1.332×10^{-4}
0.0000650	6.50	5	6.50×10^{-5}
0.00000126	1.26	6	1.26×10^{-6}
0.0000034	3.4	6	3.4×10^{-6}
0.0000783	7.83	5	7.83×10^{-5}
0.00064	6.4	4	6.4×10^{-4}

3) Convert the following numbers from scientific notation to numbers.

Scientific Notation	Coefficient	Exponent	# of Places to Move the Decimal Point to the Right	Number
5.62×10^6	5.62	6	6	5,620,000
7.82×10^8	7.82	8	8	782,000,000
9.3×10^5	9.3	5	5	930,000
6.2×10^7	6.2	7	7	62,000,000
1.055×10^5	1.055	5	5	105,500
2.38×10^9	2.38	9	9	2,380,000,000
6.90×10^3	6.90	3	3	6,900
2.781×10^8	2.781	8	8	278,100,000
4.01×10^8	4.01	8	8	401,000,000
7.56×10^5	7.56	5	5	756,000

Dosage Calculations for Nursing Students-Second Edition

4) Convert the following decimal numbers from scientific notation to decimal numbers.

Scientific Notation	Coefficient	Exponent	# of Places to Move the Decimal Point to the Left	Decimal Number
6.05×10^{-4}	6.05	-4	4	0.000605
6.3×10^{-6}	6.3	-6	6	0.0000063
4.80×10^{-5}	4.80	-5	5	0.0000480
8.51×10^{-6}	8.51	-6	6	0.00000851
6.95×10^{-5}	6.95	-5	5	0.0000695
1.023×10^{-8}	1.023	-8	8	0.00000001023
5.01×10^{-4}	5.01	-4	4	0.000501
2.43×10^{-6}	2.43	-6	6	0.00000243
2.12×10^{-3}	2.12	-3	3	0.00212
1.65×10^{-7}	1.65	-7	7	0.000000165

Chapter 10
Metric Conversion Exercise Using DA

Problem	Given to be Converted	Conversion Factor	Units of the Answer
Example	2.5 g	1000 mg/g =	2500 mg
1	340 mL	1 L/1000 mL =	0.34 L
2	0.04 g	1000 mg/g =	40 mg
3	25 mm	1 cm/10 mm =	2.5 cm
4	2.5 dL	100 mL/dL =	250 mL
5	4.5 mg	1000 mcg/mg =	4500 mcg
6	200 mcg	1 mg/1000 mcg =	0.2 mg
7	43.5 mL	1 L/1000 mL =	0.0435 L
8	615 mg	1 g/1000 mg =	0.615 g
9	2.5 kg	1000 g/kg =	2500 g
10	1.45 g	1000 mg/g =	1450 mg
11	3 mg	1000 mcg/mg =	3000 mcg
12	585 g	1 kg/1000 g =	0.585 kg
13	75,000 mcg	1 mg/1000 mcg =	75 mg
14	25 mcg	1 mg/ 1000 mcg =	0.025 mg
15	3.5 L	1000 mL/L =	3500 mL
16	2.32 g	1000 mg/g =	2320 mg
17	500 mcg	1 mg/1000 mcg =	0.5 mg
18	3 mg	1000 mcg/mg =	3000 mcg
19	25 mL	1 L/1000 mL =	0.025 L
20	3.5 m	100 cm/m =	350 cm

Dosage Calculations for Nursing Students-Second Edition

Metric Conversion Exercise Using RP

Problem	Given	Units of the Answer	Set up Equation	Answer (Solve for x) and include units
Example	3.5 g	mg	$\dfrac{x\ mg}{3.5\ g} = \dfrac{1000\ mg}{1\ g}$	3500 mg
1	5.4 g	mg	$\dfrac{x\ mg}{5.4\ g} = \dfrac{1000\ mg}{g}$	5400 mg
2	354 mcg	mg	$\dfrac{x\ mg}{354\ mcg} = \dfrac{1\ mg}{1000\ mcg}$	0.354 mg
3	5.4 kg	g	$\dfrac{x\ g}{5.4\ kg} = \dfrac{1000\ g}{kg}$	5400 g
4	102 g	kg	$\dfrac{x\ kg}{102\ g} = \dfrac{1\ kg}{1000\ g}$	0.102 kg
5	3.5 m	cm	$\dfrac{x\ cm}{3.5\ m} = \dfrac{100\ cm}{m}$	350 cm
6	1.6 dL	L	$\dfrac{x\ L}{1.6\ dL} = \dfrac{1\ L}{10\ dL}$	0.16 L
7	250 mL	L	$\dfrac{x\ L}{250\ mL} = \dfrac{1\ L}{1000\ mL}$	0.25 L
8	4.1 g	mg	$\dfrac{x\ mg}{4.1\ g} = \dfrac{1000\ mg}{g}$	4100 mg
9	25 mcg	mg	$\dfrac{x\ mg}{25\ mcg} = \dfrac{1\ mg}{1000\ mcg}$	0.025 mg
10	6 mm	cm	$\dfrac{x\ cm}{6\ mm} = \dfrac{1\ cm}{10\ mm}$	0.6 cm
11	500 g	kg	$\dfrac{x\ kg}{500\ g} = \dfrac{1\ kg}{1000\ g}$	0.5 kg
12	3.1 L	mL	$\dfrac{x\ mL}{3.1\ L} = \dfrac{1000\ mL}{L}$	3100 mL
13	815 mcg	mg	$\dfrac{x\ mg}{815\ mcg} = \dfrac{1\ mg}{1000\ mcg}$	0.815 mg
14	8.6 kg	g	$\dfrac{x\ g}{8.6\ kg} = \dfrac{1000\ g}{kg}$	8600 kg
15	0.09 mg	mcg	$\dfrac{x\ mcg}{0.09\ mg} = \dfrac{1000\ mcg}{mg}$	90 mcg

Chapter 11
Household Conversion Exercise Using DA

Problem	Given to be Converted	Conversion Factor	Units of the Answer
Example	2 fl oz	2 tbs/fl oz =	4 tbs
1	3 cups	8 fl oz/cup =	24 fl oz
2	3 gal	4 qt/gal =	12 qt
3	24 fl oz	1 cup/8 fl oz =	3 cups
4	6 tsp	1 tbs/3 tsp =	2 tbs
5	0.5 gal	8 pt/gal =	4 pt
6	0.5 pt	16 fl oz/pt =	8 fl oz
7	3 tsp	1 tbs/3 tsp =	1 tbs
8	8 oz	1 lb/16 oz =	0.5 lb
9	0.5 qt	32 fl oz/qt =	16 fl oz
10	4 tsp	1 fl oz/6 tsp =	0.67 fl oz
11	1.5 qt	32 fl oz/qt =	48 fl oz
12	16 fl oz	1 cup/8 fl oz =	2 cups
13	4 pt	1 qt/2 pt =	2 qt
14	6 fl oz	2 tbs/fl oz =	12 tbs
15	4 tbs	1 fl oz/2 tbs =	2 fl oz
16	6 tsp	1 tbs/3 tsp =	2 tbs
17	2 gal	4 qt/gal =	8 qt
18	3 fl oz	2 tbs/fl oz =	6 tbs
19	3 tsp	1 tbs/3 tsp =	1 tbs
20	2 pt	16 fl oz/pt =	32 fl oz

Household Conversion Exercise Using RP

Problem	Given	Units of the Answer	Set up Equation	Answer (Solve for x) and include units
Example	1.5 cups	fl oz	$\dfrac{x \text{ fl oz}}{1.5 \text{ cups}} = \dfrac{8 \text{ fl oz}}{1 \text{ cup}}$	12 fl oz
1	2 fl oz	tbs	$\dfrac{x \text{ tbs}}{2 \text{ fl oz}} = \dfrac{2 \text{ tbs}}{\text{fl oz}}$	4 tbs
2	4 pt	gal	$\dfrac{x \text{ gal}}{4 \text{ pt}} = \dfrac{1 \text{ gal}}{8 \text{ pt}}$	0.5 gal
3	16 fl oz	cups	$\dfrac{x \text{ cups}}{16 \text{ fl oz}} = \dfrac{1 \text{ cup}}{8 \text{ fl oz}}$	2 cups
4	1.5 gal	pt	$\dfrac{x \text{ pt}}{1.5 \text{ gal}} = \dfrac{8 \text{ pt}}{\text{gal}}$	12 pt
5	3 cups	fl oz	$\dfrac{x \text{ fl oz}}{3 \text{ cups}} = \dfrac{8 \text{ fl oz}}{\text{cup}}$	24 fl oz
6	4 pt	fl oz	$\dfrac{x \text{ fl oz}}{4 \text{ pt}} = \dfrac{16 \text{ fl oz}}{\text{pt}}$	64 fl oz
7	6 tsp	tbs	$\dfrac{x \text{ tbs}}{6 \text{ tsp}} = \dfrac{1 \text{ tbs}}{3 \text{ tsp}}$	2 tbs
8	0.5 gal	pt	$\dfrac{x \text{ pt}}{0.5 \text{ gal}} = \dfrac{8 \text{ pt}}{\text{gal}}$	4 pt
9	3 fl oz	tbs	$\dfrac{x \text{ tbs}}{3 \text{ fl oz}} = \dfrac{2 \text{ tbs}}{\text{fl oz}}$	6 tbs
10	2 tbs	fl oz	$\dfrac{x \text{ fl oz}}{2 \text{ tbs}} = \dfrac{1 \text{ fl oz}}{2 \text{ tbs}}$	1 fl oz
11	3 tsp	tbs	$\dfrac{x \text{ tbs}}{3 \text{ tsp}} = \dfrac{1 \text{ tbs}}{3 \text{ tsp}}$	1 tbs
12	3 tbs	fl oz	$\dfrac{x \text{ fl oz}}{3 \text{ tbs}} = \dfrac{1 \text{ fl oz}}{2 \text{ tbs}}$	1.5 fl oz
13	1.5 pt	cups	$\dfrac{x \text{ cups}}{1.5 \text{ pt}} = \dfrac{2 \text{ cups}}{\text{pt}}$	3 cups
14	2 qt	pt	$\dfrac{x \text{ pt}}{2 \text{ qt}} = \dfrac{2 \text{ pt}}{\text{qt}}$	4 pt
15	8 oz	lb	$\dfrac{x \text{ lb}}{8 \text{ oz}} = \dfrac{1 \text{ lb}}{16 \text{ oz}}$	0.5 lb

Chapter 12
Metric, Household and Apothecary Conversion Exercise Using DA

Problem	Given to be Converted	Conversion Factor	Units of the Answer
Example	60 mL	1 fl oz/30 mL	2 fl oz
1	2 cups	240 mL/cup	480 mL
2	4 gr	60 mg/gr	240 mg
3	180 mL	1 fl oz/30 mL	6 fl oz
4	7 in	2.54 cm/in	17.8 cm
5	0.5 pt	480 mL/pt	240 mL
6	98 mm	1 in/25.4 mm	3.9 in
7	700 g	1 lb/454 g	1.54 lb
8	16 in	2.54 cm/in	40.6 cm
9	90 mL	1 fl oz/30 mL	3 fl oz
10	48 lb	1 kg/2.2 lb	21.8 kg
11	2.2 kg	2.2 lb/kg	4.84 lb
12	2 tbs	15 mL/tbs	30 mL
13	1.8 fl oz	30 mL/fl oz	54 mL
14	3 gr	60 mg/gr	180 mg
15	60 cm	1 in/2.54 cm	23.6 in
16	240 g	1 lb/454 g	0.53 lb
17	3.2 lb	454 g/lb	1453 g
18	3 cups	240 mL/cup	720 mL
19	740 g	1 lb/454 g	1.6 lb
20	65 lb	1 kg/2.2 lb	29.5 kg

Metric, Household and Apothecary Conversion Exercise Using RP

Problem	Given	Units of the Answer	Set up Equation	Answer (Solve for x) and include units
Example	1.5 cups	mL	$\dfrac{x \text{ mL}}{1.5 \text{ cups}} = \dfrac{240 \text{ mL}}{1 \text{ cup}}$	360 mL
1	42 kg	lb	$\dfrac{x \text{ lb}}{42 \text{ kg}} = \dfrac{2.2 \text{ lb}}{\text{kg}}$	92.4 lb
2	3 tbs	mL	$\dfrac{x \text{ mL}}{3 \text{ tbs}} = \dfrac{15 \text{ mL}}{\text{tbs}}$	45 mL
3	254 cm	in	$\dfrac{x \text{ in}}{254 \text{ cm}} = \dfrac{1 \text{ in}}{2.54}$	100 in
4	250 g	lb	$\dfrac{x \text{ lb}}{250 \text{ g}} = \dfrac{1 \text{ lb}}{454 \text{ g}}$	0.55 lb
5	68 lb	kg	$\dfrac{x \text{ kg}}{68 \text{ lb}} = \dfrac{1 \text{ kg}}{2.2 \text{ lb}}$	30.9 kg
6	10 in	cm	$\dfrac{x \text{ cm}}{10 \text{ in}} = \dfrac{2.54 \text{ cm}}{\text{in}}$	25.4 cm
7	3 gr	mg	$\dfrac{x \text{ mg}}{3 \text{ gr}} = \dfrac{60 \text{ mg}}{\text{gr}}$	180 mg
8	8 fl oz	pt	$\dfrac{x \text{ pt}}{8 \text{ fl oz}} = \dfrac{1 \text{ pt}}{16 \text{ oz}}$	0.5 pt
9	95 mm	in	$\dfrac{x \text{ in}}{95 \text{ mm}} = \dfrac{1 \text{ in}}{25.4 \text{ mm}}$	3.7 in
10	750 g	lb	$\dfrac{x \text{ lb}}{750 \text{ g}} = \dfrac{1 \text{ lb}}{454 \text{ g}}$	1.65 lb
11	120 mg	gr	$\dfrac{x \text{ gr}}{120 \text{ mg}} = \dfrac{1 \text{ gr}}{60 \text{ mg}}$	2 gr
12	2 cups	mL	$\dfrac{x \text{ mL}}{2 \text{ cups}} = \dfrac{240 \text{ mL}}{\text{cup}}$	480 mL
13	15 in	cm	$\dfrac{x \text{ cm}}{15 \text{ in}} = \dfrac{2.54 \text{ cm}}{\text{in}}$	38.1 cm
14	30 mg	gr	$\dfrac{x \text{ gr}}{30 \text{ mg}} = \dfrac{1 \text{ gr}}{60 \text{ mg}}$	0.5 gr
15	3.5 lb	oz	$\dfrac{x \text{ oz}}{3.5 \text{ lb}} = \dfrac{16 \text{ oz}}{\text{lb}}$	56 oz

Chapter 13
Pounds and Ounces Conversion Exercise

Convert the following to decimal pounds.

1) 8 lb 8 oz   8 oz (1 lb/16 oz) = 0.5 lb   8 lb + 0.5 lb = 8.5 lb

2) 12 lb 4 oz   4 oz (1 lb/16 oz) = 0.25 lb   12 lb + 0.25 lb = 12.25 lb

3) 6 lb 10 oz   10 oz (1 lb/16 oz) = 0.63 lb   6 lb + 0.63 lb = 6.63 lb

4) 7 lb 9 oz   9 oz (1 lb/16 oz) = 0.56 lb   7 lb + 0.56 lb = 7.56 lb

5) 5 lb 14 oz   14 oz (1 lb/16 oz) = 0.88 lb   5 lb + 0.88 lb = 5.88 lb

Convert the following to kilograms.

6) 14 lb 6 oz   6 oz (1 lb/16 oz) = 0.38 lb   14 lb + 0.38 lb = 14.38 lb
   14.38 lb (1 kg/2.2 lb) = 6.54 kg

7) 10 lb 5 oz   5 oz (1 lb/16 oz) = 0.31 lb   10 lb + 0.31 lb = 10.31 lb
   10.31 lb (1 kg/2.2 lb) = 4.69 kg

8) 17 lb 9 oz   9 oz (1 lb/16 oz) = 0.56 lb   17 lb + 0.56 lb = 17.56 lb
   17.56 lb (1 kg/2.2 lb) = 7.98 kg

9) 16 lb 15 oz   15 oz (1 lb/16 oz) = 0.94 lb   16 lb + 0.94 lb = 16.94 lb
   16.94 lb (1 kg/2.2 lb) = 7.7 kg

10) 21 lb 4 oz   4 oz (1 lb/16 oz) = 0.25 lb   21 lb + 0.25 lb = 21.25 lb
    21.25 lb (1 kg/2.2 lb) = 9.66 kg

Convert the following to grams.

11) 3 lb 2 oz   2 oz (1 lb/16 oz) = 0.13 lb   3 lb + 0.13 lb = 3.13 lb
    3.13 lb (454 g/ lb) = 1421 g

12) 4 lb 6 oz   6 oz (1 lb/16 oz) = 0.38 lb   4 lb + 0.38 lb = 4.38 lb
    4.38 lb (454 g/ lb) = 1989 g

13) 3 lb 9 oz   9 oz (1 lb/16 oz) = 0.56 lb   3 lb + 0.56 lb = 3.56 lb
    3.56 lb (454 g/ lb) = 1616 g

14) 5 lb 7 oz   7 oz (1 lb/16 oz) = 0.44 lb   5 lb + 0.44 lb = 5.44 lb
    5.44 lb (454 g/ lb) = 2470 g

15) 5 lb 4 oz   4 oz (1 lb/16 oz) = 0.25 lb   5 lb + 0.25 lb = 5.25 lb
    5.25 lb (454 g/ lb) = 2384 g

Chapter 14
Hours and Minutes Conversion Exercise

Convert the following decimal hours to hours and minutes. Round to the nearest minute.

1) 7.4 h	0.4 h (60 min/h) = 24 min	7 h + 24 min = 7 h 24 min
2) 3.8 h	0.8 h (60 min/h) = 48 min	3 h + 48 min = 3 h 48 min
3) 8.1 h	0.1 h (60 min/h) = 6 min	8 h + 6 min = 8 h 6 min
4) 10.6 h	0.6 h (60 min/h) = 36 min	10 h + 36 min = 10 h 36 min
5) 9.25 h	0.25 h (60 min/h) = 15 min	9 h + 15 min = 9 h 15 min
6) 4.5 h	0.5 h (60 min/h) = 30 min	4 h + 30 min = 4 h 30 min
7) 3.75 h	0.75 h (60 min/h) = 45 min	3 h + 45 min = 3 h 45 min
8) 12.33 h	0.33 h (60 min/h) = 20 min	12 h + 20 min = 12 h 20 min
9) 5.15 h	0.15 h (60 min/h) = 9 min	5 h + 9 min = 5 h 9 min
10) 8.2 h	0.2 h (60 min/h) = 12 min	8 h + 12 min = 8 h 12 min

Convert the following hours and minutes to decimal hours. Round to the nearest hundredth hour.

11) 8 h 43 min	43 min (1 h/60 min) = 0.72 h	8 h + 0.72 h = 8.72 h
12) 4 h 22 min	22 min (1 h/60 min) = 0.37 h	4 h + 0.37 h = 4.37 h
13) 1 h 13 min	13 min (1 h/60 min) = 0.22 h	1 h + 0.22 h = 1.22 h
14) 9 h 55 min	55 min (1 h/60 min) = 0.92 h	9 h + 0.92 h = 9.92 h
15) 8 h 10 min	10 min (1 h/60 min) = 0.17 h	8 h + 0.17 h = 8.17 h
16) 7 h 2 min	2 min (1 h/60 min) = 0.03 h	7 h + 0.03 h = 7.03 h
17) 1 h 15 min	15 min (1 h/60 min) = 0.25 h	1 h + 0.25 h = 1.25 h
18) 10 h 43 min	43 min (1 h/60 min) = 0.72 h	10 h + 0.72 h = 10.72 h
19) 8 h 40 min	40 min (1 h/60 min) = 0.67 h	8 h + 0.67 h = 8.67 h
20) 7 h 35 min	35 min (1 h/60 min) = 0.58 h	7 h + 0.58 h = 7.58 h

Chapter 16
Dosage Calculations Level 1 Exercise

Problem	Order (The Given)	Units of the Answer	Available (The Ratio)	Administer
Example (DA)	50 mg	mL	25 mg/mL	50 mg (1 mL/25 mg) = 2 mL
Example (RP)	50 mg	mL	25 mg/mL	$\dfrac{x\,mL}{50\,mg} = \dfrac{1\,mL}{25\,mg}$ x mL=2 mL
1-DA	75 mg	mL	25 mg/mL	75 mg (1 mL/25 mg) = 3 mL
1-RP	75 mg	mL	25 mg/mL	$\dfrac{x\,mL}{75\,mg} = \dfrac{1\,mL}{25\,mg}$ x mL=3 mL
2-DA	0.3 mg	tabs	0.1 mg tabs	0.3 mg (1 tab/0.1 mg) = 3 tabs
2-RP	0.3 mg	tabs	0.1 mg tabs	$\dfrac{x\,tabs}{0.3\,mg} = \dfrac{1\,tab}{0.1\,mg}$ x tabs=3 tabs
3-DA	75 mg	mL	150 mg/mL	75 mg (1 mL/150 mg) = 0.5 mL
3-RP	75 mg	mL	150 mg/mL	$\dfrac{x\,mL}{75\,mg} = \dfrac{1\,mL}{150\,mg}$ x mL=0.5 mL
4-DA	8 mcg	mL	10 mcg/10 mL	8 mcg (10 mL/10 mcg) = 8 mL
4-RP	8 mcg	mL	10 mcg/10 mL	$\dfrac{x\,mL}{8\,mcg} = \dfrac{10\,mL}{10\,mcg}$ x mL=8 mL
5-DA	50 mcg	mL	100 mcg/5 mL	50 mcg (5 mL/100 mcg) = 2.5 mL
5-RP	50 mcg	mL	100 mcg/5 mL	$\dfrac{x\,mL}{50\,mcg} = \dfrac{5\,mL}{100\,mcg}$ x mL=2.5 mL
6	0.125 mg	mL	0.25 mg/mL	0.125 mg (1 mL/0.25 mg) = 0.5 mL
7	150 mg	mL	300 mg/2 mL	150 mg (2 mL/300 mg) = 1 mL
8	7.5 mg	tabs	5 mg scored tabs	7.5 mg (1 tab/5 mg) = 1.5 tabs
9	3 mg	tabs	6 mg scored tabs	3 mg (1 tab/6 mg) = 0.5 tab
10	200 mcg	mL	100 mcg/mL	200 mcg (1 mL/100 mcg) = 2 mL
11	480 mg	mL	400 mg/5 mL	480 mg (5 mL/400 mg) = 6 mL
12	1 g	tabs	0.25 g tab	1 g (1 tab/0.25 g) = 4 tabs
13	50 mcg	mL	200 mcg/mL	50 mcg (1 mL/200 mcg) = 0.25 mL
14	0.25 mg	tabs	0.125 mg tabs	0.25 mg (1 tab/0.125 mg) = 2 tabs
15	1 mg	mL	10 mg/mL	1 mg (1 mL/10 mg) = 0.1 mL
16	90 mg	mL	60 mg/mL	90 mg (1 mL/60 mg) = 1.5 mL
17	150 mg	mL	100 mg/mL	150 mg (1 mL/100 mg) = 1.5 mL
18	40 mg	mL	50 mg/mL	40 mg (1 mL/50 mg) = 0.8 mL
19	0.25 g	tabs	0.5 g scored tabs	0.25 g (1 tab/0.5 g) = 0.5 tab
20	20 mg	mL	5 mg/mL	20 mg (1 mL/5 mg) = 4 mL

Chapter 17
Dosage Calculations Level 2 Exercise

1) Your 42 YO patient has an order for 200 mg IM q 12 h. The drug is available as 100 mg/mL. How many mL will you administer per day?

$$\frac{200 \text{ mg}}{\text{dose}} \left(\frac{2 \text{ doses}}{\text{day}}\right)\left(\frac{1 \text{ mL}}{100 \text{ mg}}\right) = \frac{4 \text{ mL}}{\text{day}}$$

2) The physician has ordered 1000 mg/day PO divided into 2 doses of a drug which is available in 250 mg capsules. How many capsules will you administer per dose?

$$\frac{1000 \text{ mg}}{\text{day}} \left(\frac{1 \text{ day}}{2 \text{ doses}}\right)\left(\frac{1 \text{ cap}}{250 \text{ mg}}\right) = \frac{2 \text{ caps}}{\text{dose}}$$

3) Your patient has an order for 600 mg/day IV divided into 3 doses. You have available a 10 mL vial containing 500 mg of the drug. How many mL will you administer per dose?

$$\frac{600 \text{ mg}}{\text{day}} \left(\frac{1 \text{ day}}{3 \text{ doses}}\right)\left(\frac{10 \text{ mL}}{500 \text{ mg}}\right) = \frac{4 \text{ mL}}{\text{dose}}$$

4) Your pediatric patient will be going home with a 150 mL bottle of amoxicillin 125 mg/5 mL with instructions for 5 mL to be given PO q 8 h. How many days will the bottle last?

$$150 \text{ mL} \left(\frac{1 \text{ dose}}{5 \text{ mL}}\right)\left(\frac{1 \text{ day}}{3 \text{ doses}}\right) = 10 \text{ days}$$

5) The NP has ordered 100 mg IM b.i.d. of a drug which is available in 5 mL vials labeled 50 mg/mL. How many mL will you administer per dose?

$$\frac{100 \text{ mg}}{\text{dose}} \left(\frac{1 \text{ mL}}{50 \text{ mg}}\right) = \frac{2 \text{ mL}}{\text{dose}}$$

On problems like this, it is fine to leave out "dose" and just do the problem as follows.

$$100 \text{ mg} \left(\frac{1 \text{ mL}}{50 \text{ mg}}\right) = 2 \text{ mL}$$

6) The order is 500 mcg IV. On hand you have a 2 mL vial containing 1 mg/mL. How many mL will you administer?

$$500 \text{ mcg} \left(\frac{1 \text{ mL}}{1 \text{ mg}}\right)\left(\frac{1 \text{ mg}}{1000 \text{ mcg}}\right) = 0.5 \text{ mL}$$

7) Your patient has an order for 800 mg/day IV divided into 4 doses. You have available a 5 mL vial containing 1 g of the drug. How many mL will you administer per dose?

$$\frac{800 \text{ mg}}{\text{day}} \left(\frac{1 \text{ day}}{4 \text{ doses}}\right)\left(\frac{5 \text{ mL}}{1 \text{ g}}\right)\left(\frac{1 \text{ g}}{1000 \text{ mg}}\right) = \frac{1 \text{ mL}}{\text{dose}}$$

8) Your 32 YO patient who weighs 188 lb has an order for 100 mg/day IV divided into 4 doses. The drug is available in 10 mL vials containing 50 mg/mL. How many mL will you administer per dose?

$$\frac{100 \text{ mg}}{\text{day}} \left(\frac{1 \text{ day}}{4 \text{ doses}}\right)\left(\frac{1 \text{ mL}}{50 \text{ mg}}\right) = \frac{0.5 \text{ mL}}{\text{dose}}$$

9) You have an order to administer a 400 mg dose IM of a drug which is available in 10 mL vials containing 1 g. How many mL will you administer?

$$400 \text{ mg} \left(\frac{10 \text{ mL}}{1 \text{ g}}\right)\left(\frac{1 \text{ g}}{1000 \text{ mg}}\right) = 4 \text{ mL}$$

10) You have an order for 0.25 mg of levothyroxine which is available in 125 mcg scored tablets. How many tablets will you administer?

$$0.25 \text{ mg} \left(\frac{1 \text{ tab}}{125 \text{ mcg}}\right)\left(\frac{1000 \text{ mcg}}{\text{mg}}\right) = 2 \text{ tabs}$$

Chapter 18
Dosage Calculations Level 3 Exercise

1) A 164 lb patient with atrial fibrillation is to receive an initial IV bolus of verapamil 0.1 mg/kg over at least 2 minutes. The drug is available in 4 mL vials containing 2.5 mg/mL. How many mL will you administer?

$$\frac{0.1 \text{ mg}}{\text{kg}}\left(\frac{164 \text{ lb}}{1}\right)\left(\frac{1 \text{ kg}}{2.2 \text{ lb}}\right)\left(\frac{1 \text{ mL}}{2.5 \text{ mg}}\right) = 3 \text{ mL}$$

2) A 6 YO 46 lb child with acute otitis media (AOM) is to receive oral amoxicillin 80 mg/kg/day divided every 12 hours. The amoxicillin is available in 75 mL bottles containing 400 mg/5 mL. How many mL will you administer per dose?

$$\frac{80 \text{ mg}}{\text{kg day}}\left(\frac{46 \text{ lb}}{1}\right)\left(\frac{1 \text{ kg}}{2.2 \text{ lb}}\right)\left(\frac{1 \text{ day}}{2 \text{ doses}}\right)\left(\frac{5 \text{ mL}}{400 \text{ mg}}\right) = \frac{10.5 \text{ mL}}{\text{dose}}$$

3) A 4 YO 36 lb child with hypertension has be ordered furosemide 1 mg/kg/dose PO twice daily. Furosemide oral solution is available in 60 mL bottles containing 10 mg/mL. How many mL will you administer each dose?

$$\frac{1 \text{ mg}}{\text{kg dose}}\left(\frac{36 \text{ lb}}{1}\right)\left(\frac{1 \text{ kg}}{2.2 \text{ lb}}\right)\left(\frac{1 \text{ mL}}{10 \text{ mg}}\right) = \frac{1.6 \text{ mL}}{\text{dose}}$$

4) A 7 YO child weighing 48 lb is diagnosed with bacterial sinusitis and is prescribed azithromycin 10 mg/kg PO once daily for 3 days. Azithromycin oral suspension is available in 15, 22.5 and 30 mL bottles containing 200 mg/5 mL. How many mL will you administer?

$$\frac{10 \text{ mg}}{\text{kg}}\left(\frac{48 \text{ lb}}{1}\right)\left(\frac{1 \text{ kg}}{2.2 \text{ lb}}\right)\left(\frac{5 \text{ mL}}{200 \text{ mg}}\right) = 5.5 \text{ mL}$$

5) A 68 YO 173 lb patient diagnosed with an M. chelonae infection has an order for amikacin 15 mg/kg IV once daily for 2 weeks (in addition to a high dose of cefoxitin). The amikacin is available in 2 mL vials containing 500 mg. How many mL will you administer each day?

$$\frac{15 \text{ mg}}{\text{kg day}}\left(\frac{173 \text{ lb}}{1}\right)\left(\frac{1 \text{ kg}}{2.2 \text{ lb}}\right)\left(\frac{2 \text{ mL}}{500 \text{ mg}}\right) = \frac{4.7 \text{ mL}}{\text{day}}$$

6) A 125 lb patient is to receive a single IV dose of ondansetron 0.15 mg/kg, in addition to other drugs, for prevention of chemotherapy-induced nausea and vomiting. Ondansetron is available in a 20 mL MDV of 2 mg/mL. How many mL will you administer?

$$\frac{0.15 \text{ mg}}{\text{kg}}\left(\frac{125 \text{ lb}}{1}\right)\left(\frac{1 \text{ kg}}{2.2 \text{ lb}}\right)\left(\frac{1 \text{ mL}}{2 \text{ mg}}\right) = 4.3 \text{ mL}$$

7) A 74 kg male diagnosed with bacterial meningitis has an order for gentamicin 5 mg/kg/day IV in divided doses every 8 hours. How many mg will you administer for each dose?

$$\frac{5 \text{ mg}}{\text{kg day}}\left(\frac{74 \text{ kg}}{1}\right)\left(\frac{1 \text{ day}}{3 \text{ doses}}\right) = \frac{123 \text{ mg}}{\text{dose}}$$

8) Your 54 YO 162 lb, 5 ft 8 in female patient diagnosed with advanced bladder cancer has been prescribed ifosfamide 1500 mg/m²/day IV for 5 days. You calculate the BSA using the Mosteller method as being 1.88 m². Ifosfamide is available in 60 mL vials containing 3 g of drug. How many mL will you administer each day?

$$\frac{1500 \text{ mg}}{\text{m}^2 \text{ day}}\left(\frac{1.88 \text{ m}^2}{1}\right)\left(\frac{60 \text{ mL}}{3 \text{ g}}\right)\left(\frac{1 \text{ g}}{1000 \text{ mg}}\right) = \frac{56.4 \text{ mL}}{\text{day}}$$

9) Drug abc has the following dosing guidelines:

Initiate therapy at 6-8 mg/kg/day IV once daily for 2 days, then decrease dosage by 25% for days 3 and 4, then discontinue. The prescriber has ordered an initial dose of 7 mg/kg/day IV for a 48 YO 189 lb male. The drug is available in 10 mL vials labeled 100 mg/mL.

a) How many mL will you administer on day 1?

$$\frac{7 \text{ mg}}{\text{kg day}} \left(\frac{189 \text{ lb}}{1}\right)\left(\frac{1 \text{ kg}}{2.2 \text{ lb}}\right)\left(\frac{1 \text{ mL}}{100 \text{ mg}}\right) = \frac{6 \text{ mL}}{\text{day}}$$

b) How many mL will you administer on day 3? (Assume patient's weight has not changed.)

$$\frac{6 \text{ mL}}{\text{day}} \left(\frac{0.75}{1}\right) = \frac{4.5 \text{ mL}}{\text{day}}$$

10) A 52 kg adult male diagnosed with sepsis has been prescribed IV ampicillin 150 mg/kg/day divided every 4 hours. How many mg will the patient receive each dose?

$$\frac{150 \text{ mg}}{\text{kg day}} \left(\frac{52 \text{ kg}}{1}\right)\left(\frac{1 \text{ day}}{6 \text{ doses}}\right) = \frac{1300 \text{ mg}}{\text{dose}}$$

Chapter 19
BSA Calculation Exercise

Calculate the BSA in m² for the following individuals.

1) An adult male weighing 83 kg and 185 cm tall.

$$\sqrt{\frac{83 \times 185}{3600}} = 2.07 \text{ m}^2$$

2) An adult female weighing 120 lb and 5 ft 6 in tall.

$$\sqrt{\frac{120 \times 66}{3131}} = 1.59 \text{ m}^2$$

3) A 13-month-old girl weighing 23 lb and 31 in tall.

$$\sqrt{\frac{23 \times 31}{3131}} = 0.48 \text{ m}^2$$

4) A 16 YO female weighing 54 kg and 164 cm tall.

$$\sqrt{\frac{54 \times 164}{3600}} = 1.57 \text{ m}^2$$

5) An adult male weighing 238 lb and 6 ft 6 in tall.

$$\sqrt{\frac{238 \times 78}{3131}} = 2.43 \text{ m}^2$$

6) A 6 YO boy weighing 20 kg and 115 cm tall.

$$\sqrt{\frac{20 \times 115}{3600}} = 0.80 \text{ m}^2$$

7) An adult male weighing 164 lb and 5 ft 9 in tall.

$$\sqrt{\frac{164 \times 69}{3131}} = 1.90 \text{ m}^2$$

8) An adult female weighing 112 lb and 4 ft 10 in tall.

$$\sqrt{\frac{112 \times 58}{3131}} = 1.44 \text{ m}^2$$

9) An adult male weighing 173 lb and 6 ft tall.

$$\sqrt{\frac{173 \times 72}{3131}} = 1.99 \text{ m}^2$$

10) An adult female weighing 148 lb and 5 ft 1 in tall.

$$\sqrt{\frac{148 \times 61}{3131}} = 1.70 \text{ m}^2$$

Calculate the following:

11) A 54 YO male patient who weighs 184 lb and is 5 ft 10 in tall is being treated for refractory multiple myeloma and will be placed on a carfilzomib 20/27 mg/m² IV twice weekly regimen. Cycle 1 of the regimen will be 20 mg/m² infused over 10 minutes on days 1 and 2, followed by 27 mg/m² over 10 minutes on days 8, 9, 15, and 16 of a 28-day treatment cycle.

a) Calculate the patient's BSA.

$$\sqrt{\frac{184 \times 70}{3131}} = 2.03 \text{ m}^2$$

b) Calculate the dose in mg the patient will receive on days 1 and 2.

$$\frac{20 \text{ mg}}{\text{m}^2} \left(\frac{2.03 \text{ m}^2}{1} \right) = 40.6 \text{ mg}$$

c) Calculate the dose the patient will receive on days 8, 9, 15, and 16.

$$\frac{27 \text{ mg}}{\text{m}^2} \left(\frac{2.03 \text{ m}^2}{1} \right) = 54.8 \text{ mg}$$

12) A 68 YO male patient who weighs 155 lb and is 5 ft 9 in tall is being treated for acute myeloid leukemia with IV idarubicin 12 mg/m²/day for 3 days (in combination with cytarabine).

a) Calculate the patient's BSA.

$$\sqrt{\frac{155 \times 69}{3131}} = 1.85 \text{ m}^2$$

b) Calculate the daily dose in mg for this patient.

$$\frac{12\text{ mg}}{m^2\text{ day}}\left(\frac{1.85\text{ m}^2}{1}\right)=\frac{22.2\text{ mg}}{\text{day}}$$

13) A 10 YO 74 lb boy who is 4 ft 7 in tall is to receive IV topotecan 2.4 mg/m² once daily for 7 days for treatment of acute lymphoblastic leukemia.

a) Calculate the patient's BSA.

$$\sqrt{\frac{74\text{ X }55}{3131}}=1.14\text{ m}^2$$

b) Calculate the daily dose in mg for this patient.

$$\frac{2.4\text{ mg}}{m^2\text{ day}}\left(\frac{1.14\text{ m}^2}{1}\right)=\frac{2.7\text{ mg}}{\text{day}}$$

14) A 10 YO male child who weighs 30 kg and is 137 cm tall will start the BEACOPP regimen for treatment of Hodgkin lymphoma. Oral prednisone is part of the regimen dosed at 40 mg/m²/day in 2 divided doses on days 0 to 13.

a) Calculate the patient's BSA.

$$\sqrt{\frac{30\text{ X }137}{3600}}=1.07\text{ m}^2$$

b) How many milligrams of prednisone will the patient receive per dose?

$$\frac{40\text{ mg}}{m^2\text{ day}}\left(\frac{1.07\text{ m}^2}{1}\right)\left(\frac{1\text{ day}}{2\text{ doses}}\right)=\frac{21.4\text{ mg}}{\text{dose}}$$

Chapter 20
Pediatric Dosage Calculations Exercise

1) The recommended oral dosage of penicillin V potassium (penicillin VK) to treat community acquired pneumonia (CAP) in infants, children and adolescents is 50 to 75 mg/kg/day in 3 to 4 divided doses (with a maximum daily dose of 2000 mg) for 7-10 days. A 4 YO 36 lb child has been prescribed penicillin VK oral solution 250 mg PO q.i.d. for 10 days. The drug is available as 250 mg/5 mL.

1) What is the recommended range in mg/dose for this child when dosed q.i.d. (4 times daily)?

$$\frac{50 \text{ mg}}{\text{kg day}} \left(\frac{36 \text{ lb}}{1}\right)\left(\frac{1 \text{ kg}}{2.2 \text{ lb}}\right)\left(\frac{1 \text{ day}}{4 \text{ doses}}\right) = \frac{205 \text{ mg}}{\text{dose}}$$

$$\frac{75 \text{ mg}}{\text{kg day}} \left(\frac{36 \text{ lb}}{1}\right)\left(\frac{1 \text{ kg}}{2.2 \text{ lb}}\right)\left(\frac{1 \text{ day}}{4 \text{ doses}}\right) = \frac{307 \text{ mg}}{\text{dose}}$$

Answer: 205 to 307 mg/dose

2) Is the prescribed dosage within the recommended range for CAP?

Yes: 250 mg/dose is between 205 and 307 mg/dose.

3) What is the range in mL/dose for this child?

$$\frac{205 \text{ mg}}{\text{dose}}\left(\frac{5 \text{ mL}}{250 \text{ mg}}\right) = \frac{4.1 \text{ mL}}{\text{dose}}$$

$$\frac{307 \text{ mg}}{\text{dose}}\left(\frac{5 \text{ mL}}{250 \text{ mg}}\right) = \frac{6.1 \text{ mL}}{\text{dose}}$$

Answer: 4.1 to 6.1 mL/dose

4) How many mL/dose would the child receive for the prescribed dosage?

$$250 \text{ mg}\left(\frac{5 \text{ mL}}{250 \text{ mg}}\right) = 5 \text{ mL}$$

The recommended oral dosage of cephalexin to treat community acquired pneumonia caused by S. aureus (methicillin-susceptible) in children and adolescents is 75 to 100 mg/kg/day in 3 to 4 divided doses (with a maximum daily dose of 4000 mg/day) for 7-10 days. A 4 YO child weighing 34 lb has been prescribed 500 mg PO q 8 h for 7 days. The drug is available as 250 mg/5 mL.

5) What is the recommended range in mg/dose for this child when dosed q 8 h?

$$\frac{75 \text{ mg}}{\text{kg day}}\left(\frac{34 \text{ lb}}{1}\right)\left(\frac{1 \text{ kg}}{2.2 \text{ lb}}\right)\left(\frac{1 \text{ day}}{3 \text{ doses}}\right) = \frac{386 \text{ mg}}{\text{dose}}$$

$$\frac{100 \text{ mg}}{\text{kg day}}\left(\frac{34 \text{ lb}}{1}\right)\left(\frac{1 \text{ kg}}{2.2 \text{ lb}}\right)\left(\frac{1 \text{ day}}{3 \text{ doses}}\right) = \frac{515 \text{ mg}}{\text{dose}}$$

Answer: 386 to 515 mg/dose

6) Is the prescribed dosage within the recommended range for this diagnosis?

Yes. 500 mg/dose is between 386 and 515 mg/dose.

7) What is the range in mL/dose for this child?

$$\frac{386 \text{ mg}}{\text{dose}} \left(\frac{5 \text{ mL}}{250 \text{ mg}}\right) = \frac{7.7 \text{ mL}}{\text{dose}}$$

$$\frac{515 \text{ mg}}{\text{dose}} \left(\frac{5 \text{ mL}}{250 \text{ mg}}\right) = \frac{10.3 \text{ mL}}{\text{dose}}$$

Answer: 7.7 to 10.3 mL/dose

8) How many mL/dose would the child receive for the prescribed dosage?

$$500 \text{ mg} \left(\frac{5 \text{ mL}}{250 \text{ mg}}\right) = 10 \text{ mL}$$

The recommended oral dosage for diphenhydramine is 5 mg/kg/day divided into 3-4 doses, with a maximum daily dose of 300 mg/day, when treating allergies in infants, children and adolescents. An 8 YO 57 lb male child has been prescribed 30 mg PO q 6 h. Diphenhydramine is available as an oral solution containing 12.5 mg/5 mL.

9) Is this a reasonable dosage for this child?

$$\frac{5 \text{ mg}}{\text{kg day}} \left(\frac{57 \text{ lb}}{1}\right)\left(\frac{1 \text{ kg}}{2.2 \text{ lb}}\right)\left(\frac{1 \text{ day}}{4 \text{ doses}}\right) = \frac{32.4 \text{ mg}}{\text{dose}}$$

Yes, 30 mg is just a little below the recommended dose.

10) How many mL/dose will the child receive?

$$30 \text{ mg} \left(\frac{5 \text{ mL}}{12.5 \text{ mg}}\right) = 12 \text{ mL}$$

The dosing guidelines for oral morphine sulfate solution for treating moderate to severe acute pain in infants >6 months, children and adolescents who are <50 kg is 0.2 to 0.5 mg/kg/dose every 3 to 4 hours as needed and for children and adolescents 50 kg and over it is 15 to 20 mg every 3 to 4 hours as needed. Morphine sulfate oral solution 2 mg/mL and 4 mg/mL is available.

11) Using the above information, what is the normal mg/dose range for a 10 YO 32 kg male child?

$$\frac{0.2 \text{ mg}}{\text{kg dose}} \left(\frac{32 \text{ kg}}{1}\right) = \frac{6.4 \text{ mg}}{\text{dose}}$$

$$\frac{0.5 \text{ mg}}{\text{kg dose}} \left(\frac{32 \text{ kg}}{1}\right) = \frac{16 \text{ mg}}{\text{dose}}$$

Answer: 6.4 to 16 mg/dose

12) What is the normal mL/dose range using the 2 mg/mL solution for a 13-month-old 20 lb child?

$$\frac{0.2 \text{ mg}}{\text{kg dose}} \left(\frac{20 \text{ lb}}{1}\right) \left(\frac{1 \text{ kg}}{2.2 \text{ lb}}\right) \left(\frac{1 \text{ mL}}{2 \text{ mg}}\right) = \frac{0.91 \text{ mL}}{\text{dose}}$$

$$\frac{0.5 \text{ mg}}{\text{kg dose}} \left(\frac{20 \text{ lb}}{1}\right) \left(\frac{1 \text{ kg}}{2.2 \text{ lb}}\right) \left(\frac{1 \text{ mL}}{2 \text{ mg}}\right) = \frac{2.3 \text{ mL}}{\text{dose}}$$

Answer: 0.91 to 2.3 mL/dose

13) The prescriber has ordered 2 mL/dose of the 4 mg/mL morphine sulfate solution for your 4 YO patient who weighs 18 kg. Is this dose within the dosing guidelines?

$$\frac{2 \text{ mL}}{\text{dose}} \left(\frac{4 \text{ mg}}{\text{mL}}\right) \left(\frac{1}{18 \text{ kg}}\right) = \frac{0.44 \text{ mg}}{\text{kg dose}}$$

Answer: Yes. 0.44 mg/kg/dose is between 0.2 and 0.5 mg/kg/dose.

14) The prescriber, who wants to order the highest recommended dose of oral morphine sulfate solution for a 14 kg 3 YO child, has ordered 3.9 mL of the 4 mg/mL solution. Is this the correct dose? If not, what is a possible cause of the error?

$$\frac{3.9 \text{ mL}}{\text{dose}} \left(\frac{4 \text{ mg}}{\text{mL}}\right) \left(\frac{1}{14 \text{ kg}}\right) = \frac{1.1 \text{ mg}}{\text{kg dose}}$$

Answer: No, this dose is too high. The prescriber may have used the child's weight in pounds and not converted to kilograms.

Chapter 21
Pediatric Maintenance Fluid Replacement Calculations

Weight	24 Hour Fluid Requirement
Infants 3.5 to 10 kg	100 mL/kg
Children 11-20 kg	1000 mL + 50 mL/kg for every kg over 10
For children > 20 kg	1500 mL + 20 mL/kg for every kg over 20, up to a maximum of 2400 mL daily.

Use the above table in the following calculations. Round to the nearest mL and nearest mL/h.

1) Calculate the daily maintenance fluid requirement for an NPO child weighing 42.5 kg.

1500 mL + 22.5 kg (20 mL/kg) = 1500 mL + 450 mL = 1950 mL

2) Calculate the daily maintenance fluid requirement for an NPO child weighing 24 kg.

1500 mL + 4 kg (20 mL/kg) = 1500 mL + 80 mL = 1580 mL

3) Calculate the daily maintenance fluid requirement for an NPO child weighing 13 kg.

1000 mL + 3 kg (50 mL/kg) = 1000 mL + 150 mL = 1150 mL

4) Calculate the daily maintenance fluid requirement for an NPO child weighing 9.5 kg.

9.5 kg (100 mL/kg) = 950 mL

5) A 37 kg NPO child is on 70% fluid maintenance (70% of the calculated amount in the above table). At what rate will you set the infusion pump?

1500 mL + 17 kg (20 mL/kg) = 1500 mL + 340 mL = 1840 mL

0.70 (1840 mL) = 1288 mL

1288 mL/24 h = 54 mL/h

6) What is the daily maintenance fluid requirement for an NPO child on 70% fluid maintenance who weighs 17.5 kg? At what rate will you set the infusion pump?

1000 mL + 7.5 kg (50 mL/kg) = 1000 mL + 375 mL = 1375 mL

0.70 (1375 mL) = 963 mL

963 mL/24 h = 40 mL/h

7) What is the daily maintenance fluid requirement for an NPO child on 70% fluid maintenance who weighs 34 kg?

1500 mL + 14 kg (20 mL/kg) = 1500 mL + 280 mL = 1780 mL

0.70 (1780 mL) = 1246 mL

8) Calculate the daily maintenance fluid requirement for an NPO child weighing 30.5 kg.

1500 mL + 10.5 kg (20 mL/kg) = 1500 mL + 210 mL = 1710 mL

9) Calculate the infusion rate to deliver daily maintenance fluids to an NPO child weighing 36 kg.

1500 mL + 16 kg (20 mL/kg) = 1500 mL + 320 mL = 1820 mL

1820 mL/24 h = 76 mL/h

10) What is the daily maintenance fluid requirement for an NPO child on 70% fluid maintenance who weighs 43 kg? At what rate will you set the infusion pump?

1500 mL + 23 kg (20 mL/kg) = 1500 mL + 460 mL = 1960 mL

0.70 (1960 mL) = 1372 mL

1372 mL/24 h = 57 mL/h

11) At what rate will you set the infusion pump to deliver maintenance fluids to a 17 kg NPO child who is on 70% fluid maintenance?

1000 mL + 7 kg (50 mL/kg) = 1000 mL + 350 mL = 1350 mL

0.70 (1350 mL) = 945 mL

945 mL/24 h = 39 mL/h

12) Calculate the daily maintenance fluid requirement for an NPO child weighing 29 kg.

1500 mL + 9 kg (20 mL/kg) = 1500 mL + 180 mL = 1680 mL

Chapter 23
IV Flow Rate Calculations Level 1 Exercise

Round all drops/min to the nearest drop. Round all mL/hour rates for the infusion pump to the nearest tenth mL/hour.

Calculate the flow rate in mL/h.

1) 1000 mL infused over 5 hours.

$$\frac{1000 \text{ mL}}{5 \text{ h}} = \frac{200 \text{ mL}}{\text{h}}$$

2) 500 mL infused over 7 hours 30 minutes.

$$\frac{500 \text{ mL}}{7.5 \text{ h}} = \frac{66.7 \text{ mL}}{\text{h}}$$

3) 500 mL infused over 5 hours 30 minutes.

$$\frac{500 \text{ mL}}{5.5 \text{ h}} = \frac{90.9 \text{ mL}}{\text{h}}$$

4) 1000 mL infused over 8 hours.

$$\frac{1000 \text{ mL}}{8 \text{ h}} = \frac{125 \text{ mL}}{\text{h}}$$

5) 250 mL infused over 45 minutes.

$$\frac{250 \text{ mL}}{45 \text{ min}} \left(\frac{60 \text{ min}}{\text{h}}\right) = \frac{333.3 \text{ mL}}{\text{h}}$$

Or

$$\frac{250 \text{ mL}}{0.75 \text{ h}} = \frac{333.3 \text{ mL}}{\text{h}}$$

Calculate the flow rate in drops/min.

6) 1000 mL infused over 10 hours 30 minutes with a drop factor of 60 (60 gtts/mL).

$$\frac{1000 \text{ mL}}{10.5 \text{ h}} \left(\frac{1 \text{ h}}{60 \text{ min}}\right) \left(\frac{60 \text{ gtts}}{\text{mL}}\right) = \frac{95 \text{ gtts}}{\text{min}}$$

7) 500 mL infused over 90 minutes with a drop factor of 10.

$$\frac{500 \text{ mL}}{90 \text{ min}} \left(\frac{10 \text{ gtts}}{\text{mL}}\right) = \frac{56 \text{ gtts}}{\text{min}}$$

8) 1000 mL infused over 5 hours with a drop factor of 15.

$$\frac{1000 \text{ mL}}{5 \text{ h}} \left(\frac{1 \text{ h}}{60 \text{ min}}\right) \left(\frac{15 \text{ gtts}}{\text{mL}}\right) = \frac{50 \text{ gtts}}{\text{min}}$$

9) 250 mL infused over 2 hours with a microdrip set (60 gtts/mL).

$$\frac{250 \text{ mL}}{2 \text{ h}} \left(\frac{1 \text{ h}}{60 \text{ min}}\right) \left(\frac{60 \text{ gtts}}{\text{mL}}\right) = \frac{125 \text{ gtts}}{\text{min}}$$

10) 500 mL infused over 4 hours 15 minutes with a drop factor of 20.

$$\frac{500 \text{ mL}}{4.25 \text{ h}}\left(\frac{1 \text{ h}}{60 \text{ min}}\right)\left(\frac{20 \text{ gtts}}{\text{mL}}\right) = \frac{39 \text{ gtts}}{\text{min}}$$

Calculate the length of time in hours and minutes, rounded to the nearest minute, required to infuse the following:

11) 1000 mL at 63 mL/h.

$$1000 \text{ mL}\left(\frac{1 \text{ h}}{63 \text{ mL}}\right) = 15.87 \text{ h} = 15 \text{ h } 52 \text{ min}$$

12) 250 mL at 30 gtts/min with a drop factor of 20.

$$250 \text{ mL}\left(\frac{1 \text{ min}}{30 \text{ gtts}}\right)\left(\frac{20 \text{ gtts}}{\text{mL}}\right) = 167 \text{ min} = 2 \text{ h } 47 \text{ min}$$

13) 1000 mL at 80 mL/h.

$$1000 \text{ mL}\left(\frac{1 \text{ h}}{80 \text{ mL}}\right) = 12.5 \text{ h} = 12 \text{ h } 30 \text{ min}$$

14) 1000 mL at 50 gtts/min with a drop factor of 10.

$$1000 \text{ mL}\left(\frac{1 \text{ min}}{50 \text{ gtts}}\right)\left(\frac{10 \text{ gtts}}{\text{mL}}\right) = 200 \text{ min} = 3 \text{ h } 20 \text{ min}$$

15) 500 mL at 43 gtts/min with a drop factor of 10.

$$500 \text{ mL}\left(\frac{1 \text{ min}}{43 \text{ gtts}}\right)\left(\frac{10 \text{ gtts}}{\text{mL}}\right) = 116 \text{ min} = 1 \text{ h } 56 \text{ min}$$

Calculate the volume infused in the following scenarios. Round to the nearest mL.

16) Infusion rate of 60 mL per hour for 1 hour 15 min.

$$1.25 \text{ h}\left(\frac{60 \text{ mL}}{\text{h}}\right) = 75 \text{ mL}$$

17) Infusion rate of 38 mL/h for 90 min.

$$1.5 \text{ h}\left(\frac{38 \text{ mL}}{\text{h}}\right) = 57 \text{ mL}$$

18) Infusion rate of 67 mL/h for 2 hours 30 min.

$$2.5 \text{ h}\left(\frac{67 \text{ mL}}{\text{h}}\right) = 168 \text{ mL}$$

19) Infusion rate of 40 gtts/min, drop factor 20, for 6 hours 45 min.

$$6.75 \text{ h}\left(\frac{40 \text{ gtts}}{\text{min}}\right)\left(\frac{60 \text{ min}}{\text{h}}\right)\left(\frac{1 \text{ mL}}{20 \text{ gtts}}\right) = 810 \text{ mL}$$

20) Infusion rate of 28 gtts/min, drop factor 20, for 4 hours 30 min.

$$4.5 \text{ h}\left(\frac{28 \text{ gtts}}{\text{min}}\right)\left(\frac{60 \text{ min}}{\text{h}}\right)\left(\frac{1 \text{ mL}}{20 \text{ gtts}}\right) = 378 \text{ mL}$$

Chapter 24
IV Flow Rate Calculations Level 2 Exercise

Round all drops/min to the nearest drop. Round all mL/hour rates for the infusion pump to the nearest tenth mL/hour.

1) Mrs. Wilson, who has been diagnosed with acute decompensated heart failure, has an order for nitroglycerin 10 mcg/min IV. Mrs. Wilson weighs 131 lb. The NTG is available as 100 mg/250 mL. At what rate will you set the IV infusion pump?

$$\frac{10 \text{ mcg}}{\text{min}} \left(\frac{250 \text{ mL}}{100 \text{ mg}}\right) \left(\frac{1 \text{ mg}}{1000 \text{ mcg}}\right) \left(\frac{60 \text{ min}}{h}\right) = \frac{1.5 \text{ mL}}{h}$$

2) A 42 YO female who weighs 78 kg is to receive vancomycin 2 g in 400 mL D5W at a rate of 10 mg/min. At what rate will you set the IV infusion pump?

$$\frac{10 \text{ mg}}{\text{min}} \left(\frac{400 \text{ mL}}{2 \text{ g}}\right) \left(\frac{1 \text{ g}}{1000 \text{ mg}}\right) \left(\frac{60 \text{ min}}{h}\right) = \frac{120 \text{ mL}}{h}$$

3) Your 61 YO 72 kg patient has an order for a lidocaine infusion at the rate of 20 mcg/kg/min. You have a 250 mL bag labeled "Lidocaine HCl and 5% Dextrose Injection USP". Lidocaine 2 g (8 mg/mL) is printed in big red letters in the middle of the label. What rate will you set the IV infusion pump?

$$\frac{20 \text{ mcg}}{\text{kg min}} \left(\frac{72 \text{ kg}}{1}\right) \left(\frac{1 \text{ mL}}{8 \text{ mg}}\right) \left(\frac{1 \text{ mg}}{1000 \text{ mcg}}\right) \left(\frac{60 \text{ min}}{h}\right) = \frac{10.8 \text{ mL}}{h}$$

4) A healthcare provider has ordered dobutamine 10 mcg/kg/min IV for your 65 YO patient who weighs 165 lb. The dobutamine is available as 1000 mg/250 mL. At what rate will you set the IV infusion pump?

$$\frac{10 \text{ mcg}}{\text{kg min}} \left(\frac{165 \text{ lb}}{1}\right) \left(\frac{1 \text{ kg}}{2.2 \text{ lb}}\right) \left(\frac{250 \text{ mL}}{1000 \text{ mg}}\right) \left(\frac{1 \text{ mg}}{1000 \text{ mcg}}\right) \left(\frac{60 \text{ min}}{h}\right) = \frac{11.3 \text{ mL}}{h}$$

5) Your 68 kg patient is receiving a dopamine infusion at the rate of 14 mL/h. The dopamine is mixed as 200 mg of dopamine in 250 mL of D5W. The infusion has been running for 1 hour 45 minutes. How many mcg/kg/min is the patient receiving

$$\frac{14 \text{ mL}}{h} \left(\frac{1 \text{ h}}{60 \text{ min}}\right) \left(\frac{200 \text{ mg}}{250 \text{ mL}}\right) \left(\frac{1}{68 \text{ kg}}\right) \left(\frac{1000 \text{ mcg}}{\text{mg}}\right) = \frac{2.7 \text{ mcg}}{\text{kg min}}$$

6) A 37 YO female weighing 118 lb, who is being treated for a bite wound infection, has an order for ciprofloxacin 400 mg IV every 12 hours to be infused by slow IV infusion over 60 minutes. Ciprofloxacin is available in 200 mL bags containing 400 mg. You are using an IV administration set with a drop factor of 20. How many drops/min will you administer?

$$\frac{400 \text{ mg}}{60 \text{ min}} \left(\frac{200 \text{ mL}}{400 \text{ mg}}\right) \left(\frac{20 \text{ gtts}}{\text{mL}}\right) = \frac{67 \text{ gtts}}{\text{min}}$$

7) A 160 lb patient has an order for dopamine 15 mcg/kg/min to treat heart failure. The courteous pharmacy staff sends a 250 mL bag labeled dopamine 3200 mcg/mL. At what rate will you set the IV infusion pump?

$$\frac{15 \text{ mcg}}{\text{kg min}} \left(\frac{160 \text{ lb}}{1}\right) \left(\frac{1 \text{ kg}}{2.2 \text{ lb}}\right) \left(\frac{1 \text{ mL}}{3200 \text{ mcg}}\right) \left(\frac{60 \text{ min}}{h}\right) = \frac{20.5 \text{ mL}}{h}$$

8) Your 186 lb patient in vasodilatory shock has been ordered vasopressin 0.03 units/min IV. The vasopressin is available as 20 units/100 mL. At what rate will you set the IV infusion pump?

$$\frac{0.03 \text{ units}}{\text{min}} \left(\frac{100 \text{ mL}}{20 \text{ units}}\right) \left(\frac{60 \text{ min}}{h}\right) = \frac{9 \text{ mL}}{h}$$

9) A 57 YO male weighing 72 kg, who has been diagnosed with meningitis, has an order for gentamicin 5 mg/kg/day in 3 divided doses. Each dose is to be administered over 120 minutes. The drug is available in 100 mL bags containing 125 mg. At what rate will you set the IV infusion pump?

$$\frac{5 \text{ mg}}{\text{kg day}}\left(\frac{72 \text{ kg}}{1}\right)\left(\frac{1 \text{ day}}{3 \text{ doses}}\right)\left(\frac{1 \text{ dose}}{120 \text{ min}}\right)\left(\frac{100 \text{ mL}}{125 \text{ mg}}\right)\left(\frac{60 \text{ min}}{\text{h}}\right) = \frac{48 \text{ mL}}{\text{h}}$$

Or, break it up. First calculate mg/dose.

$$\frac{5 \text{ mg}}{\text{kg day}}\left(\frac{72 \text{ kg}}{1}\right)\left(\frac{1 \text{ day}}{3 \text{ doses}}\right) = \frac{120 \text{ mg}}{\text{dose}}$$

The 120 mg will be infused over 120 min, so start with that and calculate mL/h.

$$\frac{120 \text{ mg}}{120 \text{ min}}\left(\frac{60 \text{ min}}{\text{h}}\right)\left(\frac{100 \text{ mL}}{125 \text{ mg}}\right) = \frac{48 \text{ mL}}{\text{h}}$$

10) Your 53 kg patient is experiencing angina and has been titrated up from a starting dose of 5 mcg/min to 20 mcg/min of IV nitroglycerin. The NTG is available as 100 mg/250 mL. At what rate will you set the IV infusion pump?

$$\frac{20 \text{ mcg}}{\text{min}}\left(\frac{250 \text{ mL}}{100 \text{ mg}}\right)\left(\frac{1 \text{ mg}}{1000 \text{ mcg}}\right)\left(\frac{60 \text{ min}}{\text{h}}\right) = \frac{3 \text{ mL}}{\text{h}}$$

11) A 24 lb, 11-month-old infant, in shock has an order for norepinephrine 0.1 mcg/kg/min IV. The norepinephrine is available in a concentration of 8 mcg/mL. At what rate will you set the IV infusion pump?

$$\frac{0.1 \text{ mcg}}{\text{kg min}}\left(\frac{24 \text{ lb}}{1}\right)\left(\frac{1 \text{ kg}}{2.2 \text{ lb}}\right)\left(\frac{1 \text{ mL}}{8 \text{ mcg}}\right)\left(\frac{60 \text{ min}}{\text{h}}\right) = \frac{8.2 \text{ mL}}{\text{h}}$$

12) Your 57 YO female patient, who has been diagnosed with septic shock, weighs 165 lb. She has an order for norepinephrine 0.1 mcg/kg/min IV. The pharmacy delivers a bag containing 4 mg norepinephrine in 250 mL D5NS. At what rate will you set the IV infusion pump?

$$\frac{0.1 \text{ mcg}}{\text{kg min}}\left(\frac{165 \text{ lb}}{1}\right)\left(\frac{1 \text{ kg}}{2.2 \text{ lb}}\right)\left(\frac{250 \text{ mL}}{4 \text{ mg}}\right)\left(\frac{1 \text{ mg}}{1000 \text{ mcg}}\right)\left(\frac{60 \text{ min}}{\text{h}}\right) = \frac{28.1 \text{ mL}}{\text{h}}$$

13) Your 162 lb patient in vasodilatory shock has had his vasopressin titrated up to 0.035 units/min IV. The vasopressin is available as 20 units/100 mL. What rate will you set the IV infusion pump?

$$\frac{0.035 \text{ units}}{\text{min}}\left(\frac{100 \text{ mL}}{20 \text{ units}}\right)\left(\frac{60 \text{ min}}{\text{h}}\right) = \frac{10.5 \text{ mL}}{\text{h}}$$

14) Your 66 kg patient in septic shock has been ordered norepinephrine 1.5 mcg/kg/min IV. The norepinephrine is available as 4 mg in 250 mL D5W. What rate will you set the IV infusion pump?

$$\frac{1.5 \text{ mcg}}{\text{kg min}}\left(\frac{66 \text{ kg}}{1}\right)\left(\frac{250 \text{ mL}}{4 \text{ mg}}\right)\left(\frac{1 \text{ mg}}{1000 \text{ mcg}}\right)\left(\frac{60 \text{ min}}{\text{h}}\right) = \frac{371.3 \text{ mL}}{\text{h}}$$

15) A 50 YO male weighing 62 kg is to receive tobramycin 2 mg/kg/dose IV every 8 hours for a severe infection. Each dose will be administered over 40 minutes.

a) How many mg will the patient receive each dose?

$$\left(\frac{2 \text{ mg}}{\text{kg dose}}\right)\frac{62 \text{ kg}}{1} = \frac{124 \text{ mg}}{\text{dose}}$$

b) The pharmacy sends over the appropriate dose of tobramycin in a 100 mL bag of NS. At what rate will you set the IV infusion pump?

$$\frac{100 \text{ mL}}{40 \text{ min}}\left(\frac{60 \text{ min}}{\text{h}}\right) = \frac{150 \text{ mL}}{\text{h}}$$

16) A patient who weighs 165 lb is suffering from acute hypertension and has an order to start an infusion of nitroprusside 0.4 mcg/kg/min. The pharmacy delivers a 1000 mL bag containing 50 mg nitroprusside in D5W. At what rate will you set the IV infusion pump?

$$\frac{0.4 \text{ mcg}}{\text{kg min}} \left(\frac{165 \text{ lb}}{1}\right) \left(\frac{1 \text{ kg}}{2.2 \text{ lb}}\right) \left(\frac{1000 \text{ mL}}{50 \text{ mg}}\right) \left(\frac{1 \text{ mg}}{1000 \text{ mcg}}\right) \left(\frac{60 \text{ min}}{\text{h}}\right) = \frac{36 \text{ mL}}{\text{h}}$$

17) Your 91 kg patient is receiving a dopamine infusion at the rate of 15 mL/h. The dopamine is mixed as 200 mg of dopamine in 250 mL of D5W. The infusion has been running for 1 hour 25 minutes. How many mcg/kg/min is the patient receiving?

$$\frac{15 \text{ mL}}{\text{h}} \left(\frac{1 \text{ h}}{60 \text{ min}}\right) \left(\frac{200 \text{ mg}}{250 \text{ mL}}\right) \left(\frac{1}{91 \text{ kg}}\right) \left(\frac{1000 \text{ mcg}}{\text{mg}}\right) = \frac{2.2 \text{ mcg}}{\text{kg min}}$$

18) A 9 kg, 10-month-old infant, in shock has an order for norepinephrine 0.05 mcg/kg/min IV. The norepinephrine is available in a concentration of 8 mcg/mL. At what rate will you set the IV infusion pump?

$$\frac{0.05 \text{ mcg}}{\text{kg min}} \left(\frac{9 \text{ kg}}{1}\right) \left(\frac{1 \text{ mL}}{8 \text{ mcg}}\right) \left(\frac{60 \text{ min}}{\text{h}}\right) = \frac{3.4 \text{ mL}}{\text{h}}$$

19) Your 51 kg 62 YO patient diagnosed with bradycardia has an order for epinephrine 0.3 mcg/kg/min. The efficient pharmacy sends over a bag containing 1 mg epinephrine in 250 mL D5W. At what rate will you set the IV infusion pump?

$$\frac{0.3 \text{ mcg}}{\text{kg min}} \left(\frac{51 \text{ kg}}{1}\right) \left(\frac{250 \text{ mL}}{1 \text{ mg}}\right) \left(\frac{1 \text{ mg}}{1000 \text{ mcg}}\right) \left(\frac{60 \text{ min}}{\text{h}}\right) = \frac{229.5 \text{ mL}}{\text{h}}$$

20) R.M, a 69 YO female weighing 67 kg with heart failure, has an order for a continuous IV infusion of milrinone 0.5 mcg/kg/min. Milrinone is available in 100 mL bags containing 20 mg. At what rate will you set the IV infusion pump?

$$\frac{0.5 \text{ mcg}}{\text{kg min}} \left(\frac{67 \text{ kg}}{1}\right) \left(\frac{100 \text{ mL}}{20 \text{ mg}}\right) \left(\frac{1 \text{ mg}}{1000 \text{ mcg}}\right) \left(\frac{60 \text{ min}}{\text{h}}\right) = \frac{10.1 \text{ mL}}{\text{h}}$$

Chapter 25
IV Flow Rate Adjustments Exercise

You have an order for a 500 mL bag of NS to infuse over 4 hours 30 minutes with a drop factor of 15. The bag was started at 1800. At 1900 you notice that 300 mL remain.

1) What is the initial calculated rate in gtts/min?

$$\frac{500 \text{ mL}}{4.5 \text{ h}} \left(\frac{1 \text{ h}}{60 \text{ min}}\right)\left(\frac{15 \text{ gtts}}{\text{mL}}\right) = \frac{28 \text{ gtts}}{\text{min}}$$

2) What will be the new rate in gtts/min?

$$\frac{300 \text{ mL}}{3.5 \text{ h}} \left(\frac{1 \text{ h}}{60 \text{ min}}\right)\left(\frac{15 \text{ gtts}}{\text{mL}}\right) = \frac{21 \text{ gtts}}{\text{min}}$$

3) What is the percent change?

$$\frac{21 - 28}{28} (100\%) = \frac{-7}{28} (100\%) = -25\%$$

4) Will you contact the prescriber?

Yes

You have an order for a 1000 mL bag of NS to infuse over 4 hours with a drop factor of 20. The bag was started at 0800. At 0900 you notice that 850 mL remain.

5) What is the initial calculated rate in gtts/min?

$$\frac{1000 \text{ mL}}{4 \text{ h}} \left(\frac{1 \text{ h}}{60 \text{ min}}\right)\left(\frac{20 \text{ gtts}}{\text{mL}}\right) = \frac{83 \text{ gtts}}{\text{min}}$$

6) What will be the new rate in gtts/min?

$$\frac{850 \text{ mL}}{3 \text{ h}} \left(\frac{1 \text{ h}}{60 \text{ min}}\right)\left(\frac{20 \text{ gtts}}{\text{mL}}\right) = \frac{94 \text{ gtts}}{\text{min}}$$

7) What is the percent change?

$$\frac{94 - 83}{83} (100\%) = \frac{11}{83} (100\%) = 13.3\%$$

8) Will you contact the prescriber?

No

You have an order for a 1000 mL bag of D5W to infuse over 9 hours with a drop factor of 20. The bag was started at 0800. At 1400 you notice that 400 mL remain.

9) What is the initial calculated rate in gtts/min?

$$\frac{1000 \text{ mL}}{9 \text{ h}} \left(\frac{1 \text{ h}}{60 \text{ min}}\right)\left(\frac{20 \text{ gtts}}{\text{mL}}\right) = \frac{37 \text{ gtts}}{\text{min}}$$

10) What will be the new rate in gtts/min?

$$\frac{400 \text{ mL}}{3 \text{ h}} \left(\frac{1 \text{ h}}{60 \text{ min}}\right)\left(\frac{20 \text{ gtts}}{\text{mL}}\right) = \frac{44 \text{ gtts}}{\text{min}}$$

11) What is the percent change?

$$\frac{44-37}{37}(100\%) = \frac{7}{37}(100\%) = 18.9\%$$

12) Will you contact the prescriber?

No

You have an order for a 500 mL bag of NS to infuse over 2 hours with a drop factor of 20. The bag was started at 1000. At 1030 you notice that 400 mL remain.

13) What is the initial calculated rate in gtts/min?

$$\frac{500 \text{ mL}}{2 \text{ h}} \left(\frac{1 \text{ h}}{60 \text{ min}}\right)\left(\frac{20 \text{ gtts}}{\text{mL}}\right) = \frac{83 \text{ gtts}}{\text{min}}$$

14) What will be the new rate in gtts/min?

$$\frac{400 \text{ mL}}{1.5 \text{ h}} \left(\frac{1 \text{ h}}{60 \text{ min}}\right)\left(\frac{20 \text{ gtts}}{\text{mL}}\right) = \frac{89 \text{ gtts}}{\text{min}}$$

15) What is the percent change?

$$\frac{89-83}{83}(100\%) = \frac{6}{83}(100\%) = 7.2\%$$

16) Will you contact the prescriber?

No

You have an order for a 250 mL bag of NS to infuse over 2 hours with a drop factor of 60. The bag was started at 1900. At 1930 you notice that 175 mL remain.

17) What is the initial calculated rate in gtts/min?

$$\frac{250 \text{ mL}}{2 \text{ h}} \left(\frac{1 \text{ h}}{60 \text{ min}}\right)\left(\frac{60 \text{ gtts}}{\text{mL}}\right) = \frac{125 \text{ gtts}}{\text{min}}$$

18) What will be the new rate in gtts/min?

$$\frac{175 \text{ mL}}{1.5 \text{ h}} \left(\frac{1 \text{ h}}{60 \text{ min}}\right)\left(\frac{60 \text{ gtts}}{\text{mL}}\right) = \frac{117 \text{ gtts}}{\text{min}}$$

19) What is the percent change?

$$\frac{117-125}{125}(100\%) = \frac{-8}{125}(100\%) = -6.4\%$$

20) Will you contact the prescriber?

No

Chapter 26
Heparin Infusion and Adjustment Calculations Exercise

Pt C.B, a 55 YO female weighing 165 lb, has been admitted with a diagnosis of PE and has the following heparin order:
Initial bolus: 80 units/kg (max 10,000 units)
Initial infusion: 18 units/kg/h (initial max of 1800 units/h)

1) Calculate the bolus dose in units.

$$\frac{80 \text{ units}}{\text{kg}} \left(\frac{165 \text{ lb}}{1}\right)\left(\frac{1 \text{ kg}}{2.2 \text{ lb}}\right) = 6000 \text{ units}$$

2) Calculate the bolus dose in mL.

$$6000 \text{ units} \left(\frac{1 \text{ mL}}{5000 \text{ units}}\right) = 1.2 \text{ mL}$$

3) Calculate the initial infusion rate in units/h.

$$\frac{18 \text{ units}}{\text{kg h}} \left(\frac{165 \text{ lb}}{1}\right)\left(\frac{1 \text{ kg}}{2.2 \text{ lb}}\right) = \frac{1350 \text{ units}}{h} \text{ rounded to } \frac{1400 \text{ units}}{h}$$

4) Calculate the initial infusion rate in mL/h.

$$\frac{1400 \text{ units}}{h} \left(\frac{1 \text{ mL}}{100 \text{ units}}\right) = \frac{14 \text{ mL}}{h}$$

5) The initial infusion was started at 0630. At 12:30 PM you order an anti-Xa assay and it comes back at 0.95 units/mL.

a) What course of action will you take?

Hold infusion for 60 min and decrease dosage by 3 units/kg/h to 15 units/kg/h.

b) What will the new infusion rate be in units/h?

$$\frac{15 \text{ units}}{\text{kg h}} \left(\frac{165 \text{ lb}}{1}\right)\left(\frac{1 \text{ kg}}{2.2 \text{ lb}}\right) = \frac{1125 \text{ units}}{h} \text{ rounded to } \frac{1100 \text{ units}}{h}$$

6) At 1830 another anti-Xa assay is ordered and comes back at 0.91 units/mL. What is your course of action?

Contact prescriber.

7) After contacting the prescriber after the second anti-Xa assay >9.0, you are instructed to decrease the dosage by 3 units/kg/h. What will be the new rate in units/h?

$$\frac{12 \text{ units}}{\text{kg h}} \left(\frac{165 \text{ lb}}{1}\right)\left(\frac{1 \text{ kg}}{2.2 \text{ lb}}\right) = \frac{900 \text{ units}}{h}$$

Pt Y.M, who weighs 174 lb, has been admitted with a diagnosis of unstable angina and has the following heparin order:
Initial bolus: 60 units/kg (max 5,000 units)
Initial infusion: 12 units/kg/h (initial max of 1000 units/h)

8) Calculate the bolus dose in units.

$$\frac{60 \text{ units}}{\text{kg}} \left(\frac{174 \text{ lb}}{1}\right)\left(\frac{1 \text{ kg}}{2.2 \text{ lb}}\right) = 4745 \text{ units rounded to } 4500 \text{ units}$$

9) Calculate the bolus dose in mL.

$$4500 \text{ units}\left(\frac{1 \text{ mL}}{5000 \text{ units}}\right) = 0.9 \text{ mL}$$

10) Calculate the initial infusion rate in units/h.

$$\frac{12 \text{ units}}{\text{kg h}} \left(\frac{174 \text{ lb}}{1}\right)\left(\frac{1 \text{ kg}}{2.2 \text{ lb}}\right) = \frac{949 \text{ units}}{\text{h}} \text{ rounded to } \frac{900 \text{ units}}{\text{h}}$$

11) Calculate the initial infusion rate in mL/h.

$$\frac{900 \text{ units}}{\text{h}}\left(\frac{1 \text{ mL}}{100 \text{ units}}\right) = \frac{9 \text{ mL}}{\text{h}}$$

12) The initial infusion was started at 1600. At 2200 you order an anti-Xa assay and it comes back at 0.24 units/mL.

a) What course of action will you take?

Re-bolus at 40 units/kg. Increase dosage by 2 units/kg/h to 14 units/kg/h.

b) Include all calculations.

Bolus calculations:

$$\frac{40 \text{ units}}{\text{kg}} \left(\frac{174 \text{ lb}}{1}\right)\left(\frac{1 \text{ kg}}{2.2 \text{ lb}}\right) = 3163 \text{ units rounded to } 3000 \text{ units}$$

$$3000 \text{ units}\left(\frac{1 \text{ mL}}{5000 \text{ units}}\right) = 0.6 \text{ mL}$$

Infusion calculations:

$$\frac{14 \text{ units}}{\text{kg h}} \left(\frac{174 \text{ lb}}{1}\right)\left(\frac{1 \text{ kg}}{2.2 \text{ lb}}\right) = \frac{1107 \text{ units}}{\text{h}} \text{ rounded to } \frac{1100 \text{ units}}{\text{h}}$$

$$\frac{1100 \text{ units}}{\text{h}}\left(\frac{1 \text{ mL}}{100 \text{ units}}\right) = \frac{11 \text{ mL}}{\text{h}}$$

13) At 0400 the following day another anti-Xa assay is ordered and comes back at 0.51 units/mL. Will you, or the on-duty nurse, adjust the dose? If so, what will the new infusion rate be in units/h?

No

14) At 1000 another anti-Xa assay is ordered which comes back at 0.72 units/mL.

a) What is your course of action?

Decrease dosage by 1 unit/kg/h to 13 units/kg/h.

b) Include all calculations.

$$\frac{13 \text{ units}}{\text{kg h}} \left(\frac{174 \text{ lb}}{1}\right)\left(\frac{1 \text{ kg}}{2.2 \text{ lb}}\right) = \frac{1028 \text{ units}}{\text{h}} \text{ rounded to } \frac{1000 \text{ units}}{\text{h}}$$

$$\frac{1000 \text{ units}}{\text{h}} \left(\frac{1 \text{ mL}}{100 \text{ units}}\right) = \frac{10 \text{ mL}}{\text{h}}$$

Pt T.G., who weighs 84 kg, has been admitted with a diagnosis of DVT and has the following heparin order:
Initial bolus: 80 units/kg (max 10,000 units)
Initial infusion: 18 units/kg/h (initial max of 1800 units/h)

15) Calculate the bolus dose in units.

$$\frac{80 \text{ units}}{\text{kg}} \left(\frac{84 \text{ kg}}{1}\right) = 6720 \text{ units rounded to } 6500 \text{ units}$$

16) Calculate the bolus dose in mL.

$$6500 \text{ units} \left(\frac{1 \text{ mL}}{5000 \text{ units}}\right) = 1.3 \text{ mL}$$

17) Calculate the initial infusion rate in units/h.

$$\frac{18 \text{ units}}{\text{kg h}} \left(\frac{84 \text{ kg}}{1}\right) = \frac{1512 \text{ units}}{\text{h}} \text{ rounded to } \frac{1500 \text{ units}}{\text{h}}$$

18) Calculate the initial infusion rate in mL/h.

$$\frac{1500 \text{ units}}{\text{h}} \left(\frac{1 \text{ mL}}{100 \text{ units}}\right) = \frac{15 \text{ mL}}{\text{h}}$$

19) The initial infusion was started at 1300. At 1900 you order an anti-Xa assay and it comes back at 0.77 units/mL.

a) What course of action will you take?

Decrease dosage by 1 unit/kg/h to 17 units/kg/h.

b) Include all calculations.

$$\frac{17 \text{ units}}{\text{kg h}} \left(\frac{84 \text{ kg}}{1}\right) = \frac{1428 \text{ units}}{\text{h}} \text{ rounded to } \frac{1400 \text{ units}}{\text{h}}$$

$$\frac{1400 \text{ units}}{\text{h}} \left(\frac{1 \text{ mL}}{100 \text{ units}}\right) = \frac{14 \text{ mL}}{\text{h}}$$

20) At 0100 the following day another anti-Xa assay is ordered and comes back at 0.69 units/mL. Will you, or the on-duty nurse, adjust the dose? If so, what will the new infusion rate be in units/h?

No

21) At 0700 another anti-Xa assay is ordered which comes back at 0.70 units/mL.

a) What is your course of action?

Decrease to daily monitoring (two consecutive anti-Xa levels are within therapeutic range).

b) Include all calculations.

No calculations.

Pt D.E, who weighs 79 kg, has been admitted with a diagnosis of stroke and has the following heparin order:
Initial bolus: None
Initial infusion: 12 units/kg/h (initial max of 1200 units/h)

22) Calculate the bolus dose in units.

None

23) Calculate the bolus dose in mL.

None

24) Calculate the initial infusion rate in units/h.

$$\frac{12 \text{ units}}{\text{kg h}} \left(\frac{79 \text{ kg}}{1}\right) = \frac{948 \text{ units}}{h} \text{ rounded to } \frac{900 \text{ units}}{h}$$

25) Calculate the initial infusion rate in mL/h.

$$\frac{900 \text{ units}}{h} \left(\frac{1 \text{ mL}}{100 \text{ units}}\right) = \frac{9 \text{ mL}}{h}$$

26) The initial infusion was started at 9:30 AM. At 3:30 PM you order an anti-Xa assay and it comes back at 0.55 units/mL.

a) What is your course of action?

No dosage change.

b) Include all calculations.

No calculations required.

27) At 9:30 PM another anti-Xa assay is ordered and comes back at 0.51 units/mL.

a) Will you, or the on-duty nurse, adjust the dose?

No

b) If so, what will the new infusion rate be in mL/h?

n/a

28) At 0700 another anti-Xa assay is ordered which comes back at 0.53 units/mL.

a) What is your course of action?

No dosage change. Decrease to daily monitoring.

b) When will you order the next anti-Xa?

0700 the next day.

Pt B.B., who weighs 49 kg, has been admitted with a diagnosis of PE and has the following heparin order:
Initial bolus: 80 units/kg (max 10,000 units)
Initial infusion: 18 units/kg/h (initial max of 1800 units/h)

29) Calculate the bolus dose in units.

$$\frac{80 \text{ units}}{\text{kg}} \left(\frac{49 \text{ kg}}{1}\right) = 3920 \text{ units rounded to } 4000 \text{ units}$$

30) Calculate the bolus dose in mL.

$$4000 \text{ units} \left(\frac{1 \text{ mL}}{5000 \text{ units}}\right) = 0.8 \text{ mL}$$

31) Calculate the initial infusion rate in units/h.

$$\frac{18 \text{ units}}{\text{kg h}} \left(\frac{49 \text{ kg}}{1}\right) = \frac{882 \text{ units}}{\text{h}} \text{ rounded to } \frac{900 \text{ units}}{\text{h}}$$

32) Calculate the initial infusion rate in mL/h.

$$\frac{900 \text{ units}}{\text{h}} \left(\frac{1 \text{ mL}}{100 \text{ units}}\right) = \frac{9 \text{ mL}}{\text{h}}$$

33) The initial infusion was started at 1000. At 1600 you order an anti-Xa assay and it comes back at 0.26 units/mL.

a) What course of action do you take?

Re-bolus at 40 units/kg. Increase dosage by 2 units/kg/h to 20 units/kg/h.

b) Include all calculations.

Bolus calculations:

$$\frac{40 \text{ units}}{\text{kg}} \left(\frac{49 \text{ kg}}{1}\right) = 1960 \text{ units rounded to } 2000 \text{ units}$$

$$2000 \text{ units} \left(\frac{1 \text{ mL}}{5000 \text{ units}}\right) = 0.4 \text{ mL}$$

Infusion calculations:

$$\frac{20 \text{ units}}{\text{kg h}} \left(\frac{49 \text{ kg}}{1}\right) = \frac{980 \text{ units}}{\text{h}} \text{ rounded to } \frac{1000 \text{ units}}{\text{h}}$$

$$\frac{1000 \text{ units}}{\text{h}} \left(\frac{1 \text{ mL}}{100 \text{ units}}\right) = \frac{10 \text{ mL}}{\text{h}}$$

34) At 2200 another anti-Xa assay is ordered and comes back at 0.40 units/mL.

a) Will you, or the on-duty nurse, adjust the dose?

No

b) If so, what will the new infusion rate be in units/h?

n/a

35) At 0400 the next day, another anti-Xa assay is ordered which comes back at 0.42 units/mL. What is your course of action?

No dosage change. Switch to daily monitoring.

36) Calculate the bolus dose in units. **Pt P.J., a 68 YO male weighing 83 kg has been admitted with a diagnosis of unstable angina and has the following heparin order:**
Initial bolus: 60 units/kg (max 5,000 units)
Initial infusion: 12 units/kg/h (initial max of 1000 units/h)

$$\frac{60 \text{ units}}{\text{kg}} \left(\frac{83 \text{ kg}}{1}\right) = 4980 \text{ units rounded to } 5000 \text{ units}$$

37) Calculate the bolus dose in mL.

$$5000 \text{ units} \left(\frac{1 \text{ mL}}{5000 \text{ units}}\right) = 1 \text{ mL}$$

38) Calculate the initial infusion rate in units/h.

$$\frac{12 \text{ units}}{\text{kg h}} \left(\frac{83 \text{ kg}}{1}\right) = \frac{996 \text{ units}}{\text{h}} \text{ rounded to } \frac{1000 \text{ units}}{\text{h}}$$

39) Calculate the initial infusion rate in mL/h.

$$\frac{1000 \text{ units}}{\text{h}} \left(\frac{1 \text{ mL}}{100 \text{ units}}\right) = \frac{10 \text{ mL}}{\text{h}}$$

40) The initial infusion was started at 1600. At 2200 you order an anti-Xa assay and it comes back at 0.82 units/mL.

a) What course of action will you take?

Hold infusion for 30 min. Decrease dosage by 2 units/kg/h to 10 units/kg/h.

b) Include all calculations.

$$\frac{10 \text{ units}}{\text{kg h}} \left(\frac{83 \text{ kg}}{1}\right) = \frac{830 \text{ units}}{\text{h}} \text{ rounded to } \frac{800 \text{ units}}{\text{h}}$$

$$\frac{800 \text{ units}}{\text{h}} \left(\frac{1 \text{ mL}}{100 \text{ units}}\right) = \frac{8 \text{ mL}}{\text{h}}$$

41) At 0400 the following day another anti-Xa assay is ordered and comes back at 0.75 units/mL.

a) Will you, or the on-duty nurse, adjust the dose?

Yes, decrease dosage by 1 unit/kg/h to 9 units/kg/h.

b) If so, what will the new infusion rate be in units/h?

$$\frac{9 \text{ units}}{\text{kg h}} \left(\frac{83 \text{ kg}}{1}\right) = \frac{747 \text{ units}}{\text{h}} \text{ rounded to } \frac{700 \text{ units}}{\text{h}}$$

42) At 1000 another anti-Xa assay is ordered which comes back at 0.69 units/mL. What do you do?

No dosage adjustment. Continue to monitor.

Pt A.C., who weighs 107 kg, has been admitted with a diagnosis of DVT and has the following heparin order:
Initial bolus: 80 units/kg (max 10,000 units)
Initial infusion: 18 units/kg/h (initial max of 1800 units/h)

43) Calculate the bolus dose in units.

$$\frac{80 \text{ units}}{\text{kg}} \left(\frac{107 \text{ kg}}{1}\right) = 8560 \text{ units rounded to } 8500 \text{ units}$$

44) Calculate the bolus dose in mL.

$$8500 \text{ units} \left(\frac{1 \text{ mL}}{5000 \text{ units}}\right) = 1.7 \text{ mL}$$

45) Calculate the initial infusion rate in units/h.

$$\frac{18 \text{ units}}{\text{kg h}} \left(\frac{107 \text{ kg}}{1}\right) = \frac{1926 \text{ units}}{\text{h}} \text{ max} = \frac{1800 \text{ units}}{\text{h}}$$

46) Calculate the initial infusion rate in mL/h.

$$\frac{1800 \text{ units}}{\text{h}} \left(\frac{1 \text{ mL}}{100 \text{ units}}\right) = \frac{18 \text{ mL}}{\text{h}}$$

47) The initial infusion was started at 0915. At 1515 you order an anti-Xa assay and it comes back at 0.25 units/mL.

a) What is your course of action?

Re-bolus at 40 units/kg. Increase dosage by 2 units/kg/h to 20 units/kg/h.

b) Include all calculations.

Bolus calculations:

$$\frac{40 \text{ units}}{\text{kg}} \left(\frac{107 \text{ kg}}{1}\right) = 4280 \text{ units rounded to } 4000 \text{ units}$$

$$4000 \text{ units} \left(\frac{1 \text{ mL}}{5000 \text{ units}}\right) = 0.8 \text{ mL}$$

Infusion calculations:

$$\frac{20 \text{ units}}{\text{kg h}} \left(\frac{107 \text{ kg}}{1}\right) = \frac{2140 \text{ units}}{\text{h}} \text{ rounded to } \frac{2100 \text{ units}}{\text{h}}$$

$$\frac{2100 \text{ units}}{\text{h}} \left(\frac{1 \text{ mL}}{100 \text{ units}}\right) = \frac{21 \text{ mL}}{\text{h}}$$

48) At 2115 another anti-Xa assay is ordered and comes back at 0.46 units/mL.

a) Will you, or the on-duty nurse, adjust the dose?

No

b) If so, what will the new infusion rate be in units/h?

n/a

49) At 0315 another anti-Xa assay is ordered which comes back at 0.44 units/mL. What do you do?

No dosage change. Switch to daily monitoring.

Pt W.W., who weighs 64 kg, has been admitted with a diagnosis of DVT and has the following heparin order:
Initial bolus: 80 units/kg (max 10,000 units)
Initial infusion: 18 units/kg/h (initial max of 1800 units/h)

50) Calculate the bolus dose in units.

$$\frac{80 \text{ units}}{\text{kg}}\left(\frac{64 \text{ kg}}{1}\right) = 5120 \text{ units rounded to } 5000 \text{ units}$$

51) Calculate the bolus dose in mL.

$$5000 \text{ units}\left(\frac{1 \text{ mL}}{5000 \text{ units}}\right) = 1 \text{ mL}$$

52) Calculate the initial infusion rate in units/h.

$$\frac{18 \text{ units}}{\text{kg h}}\left(\frac{64 \text{ kg}}{1}\right) = \frac{1152 \text{ units}}{\text{h}} \text{ rounded to } = \frac{1200 \text{ units}}{\text{h}}$$

53) Calculate the initial infusion rate in mL/h.

$$\frac{1200 \text{ units}}{\text{h}}\left(\frac{1 \text{ mL}}{100 \text{ units}}\right) = \frac{12 \text{ mL}}{\text{h}}$$

54) The initial infusion was started at 0600. At 1200 you order an anti-Xa assay and it comes back at 0.84 units/mL.

a) What is your course of action?

Hold infusion for 30 minutes and decrease dosage by 2 units/kg/h to 16 units/kg/h.

b) What will the new infusion rate be in units/h?

$$\frac{16 \text{ units}}{\text{kg h}}\left(\frac{64 \text{ kg}}{1}\right) = \frac{1024 \text{ units}}{\text{h}} \text{ rounded to } = \frac{1000 \text{ units}}{\text{h}}$$

55) At 1800 another anti-Xa assay is ordered and comes back at 0.74 units/mL.

a) Will you, or the on-duty nurse, adjust the dosage?

Yes, decrease by 1 unit/kg/h to 15 units/kg/h.

b) If so, what will the new infusion rate be in units/h?

$$\frac{15 \text{ units}}{\text{kg h}}\left(\frac{64 \text{ kg}}{1}\right) = \frac{960 \text{ units}}{\text{h}} \text{ rounded to } = \frac{1000 \text{ units}}{\text{h}}$$

Note: Due to rounding, the infusion rate remains at 1000 units/h. Continue to monitor.

56) At 0000 another anti-Xa assay is ordered which comes back at 0.72 units/mL.

a) Will you, or the on-duty nurse, adjust the dosage?

Yes, decrease by 1 unit/kg/h to 14 units/kg/h.

b) If so, what will the new infusion rate be in units/h?

$$\frac{14 \text{ units}}{\text{kg h}} \left(\frac{64 \text{ kg}}{1}\right) = \frac{896 \text{ units}}{\text{h}} \text{ rounded to } = \frac{900 \text{ units}}{\text{h}}$$

Chapter 27
Percent Exercise

Convert the following numbers to percents.

Problem	Number	Percent
Example	0.46	0.46 (100%) = 46%
1	0.42	0.42 (100%) = 42%
2	0.68	0.68 (100%) = 68%
3	1.392	1.392 (100%) = 139.2%
4	2.82	2.82 (100%) = 282%
5	0.005	0.005 (100%) = 0.5%
6	0.036	0.036 (100%) = 3.6%
7	1.29	1.29 (100%) = 129%
8	0.463	0.463 (100%) = 46.3%
9	0.549	0.549 (100%) = 54.9%
10	1.517	1.517 (100%) = 151.7%

Convert the following percents to numbers.

Problem	Percent	Number
Example	31%	31%/100% = 0.31
11	32.4%	32.4%/100% = 0.324
12	68%	68%/100% = 0.68
13	1.2%	1.2%/100% = 0.012
14	34.3%	34.3%/100% = 0.343
15	9.6%	9.6%/100% = 0.096
16	65.35%	65.35%/100% = 0.6535
17	1.9%	1.9%/100% = 0.019
18	3.8%	3.8%/100% = 0.038
19	1.8%	1.8%/100% = 0.018
20	0.6%	0.6%/100% = 0.006

Dosage Calculations for Nursing Students-Second Edition

Chapter 28
Percent Strength Exercise

Express the following as percent strength solutions and include the type of solution (w/w, w/v, v/v, v/w).

1) 1.5 g HC in 200 g HC ointment

$$\frac{1.5 \text{ g AI}}{200 \text{ g Oint}} 100\% = 0.75\% \text{ w/w}$$

2) 6.5 g NaCl in 1000 mL

$$\frac{6.5 \text{ g}}{1000 \text{ mL}} 100\% = 0.65\% \text{ w/v}$$

3) 25 mL ETOH in 100 mL ETOH solution

$$\frac{25 \text{ mL AI}}{100 \text{ mL Soln}} 100\% = 25\% \text{ v/v}$$

4) 2.5 mg betamethasone in 5 g betamethasone ointment

$$\frac{2.5 \text{ mg AI}}{5 \text{ g Oint}} \left(\frac{1 \text{ g AI}}{1000 \text{ mg AI}}\right) 100\% = 0.05\% \text{ w/w}$$

5) 4.5 g NaCl in 2 L

$$\frac{4.5 \text{ g}}{2 \text{ L}} \left(\frac{1 \text{ L}}{1000 \text{ mL}}\right) 100\% = 0.225\% \text{ w/v}$$

6) 25 mcg NaCl in 0.25 mL

$$\frac{25 \text{ mcg}}{0.25 \text{ mL}} \left(\frac{1 \text{ g}}{1,000,000 \text{ mcg}}\right) 100\% = 0.01\% \text{ w/v}$$

7) 500 mg NaHCO$_3$ in 200 mL

$$\frac{500 \text{ mg}}{200 \text{ mL}} \left(\frac{1 \text{ g}}{1000 \text{ mg}}\right) 100\% = 0.25\% \text{ w/v}$$

8) 5 g KCl in 200 mL

$$\frac{5 \text{ g}}{200 \text{ mL}} 100\% = 2.5\% \text{ w/v}$$

9) 10 g salicylic acid in 250 g salicylic acid cream

$$\frac{10 \text{ g AI}}{250 \text{ g Cr}} 100\% = 4\% \text{ w/w}$$

10) 10 g urea in 40 g urea ointment

$$\frac{10 \text{ g AI}}{40 \text{ g Oint}} 100\% = 25\% \text{ w/w}$$

Answer the following:

11) How many mg of lidocaine are in 300 mL of 1% lidocaine?

$$300 \text{ mL} \left(\frac{1 \text{ g}}{100 \text{ mL}}\right)\left(\frac{1000 \text{ mg}}{\text{g}}\right) = 3000 \text{ mg}$$

12) How many g of KCl are in 400 mL of 10% KCl?

$$400 \text{ mL}\left(\frac{10 \text{ g}}{100 \text{ mL}}\right) = 40 \text{ g}$$

13) How many mg of bupivacaine are in 60 mL of 0.5% bupivacaine solution?

$$60 \text{ mL}\left(\frac{0.5 \text{ g}}{100 \text{ mL}}\right)\left(\frac{1000 \text{ mg}}{\text{g}}\right) = 300 \text{ mg}$$

14) How many g of HC are in 200 g of 2.5% HC ointment?

$$200 \text{ g Oint}\left(\frac{2.5 \text{ g AI}}{100 \text{ g Oint}}\right) = 5 \text{ g AI}$$

15) How many grams of dextrose are in 2.5 L of D5W (5% dextrose in water)?

$$2.5 \text{ L}\left(\frac{5 \text{ g}}{100 \text{ mL}}\right)\left(\frac{1000 \text{ mL}}{\text{L}}\right) = 125 \text{ g}$$

16) How many mg of triamcinolone are in 45 g of 0.1% triamcinolone ointment?

$$45 \text{ g Oint}\left(\frac{0.1 \text{ g AI}}{100 \text{ g Oint}}\right)\left(\frac{1000 \text{ mg AI}}{1 \text{ g AI}}\right) = 45 \text{ mg AI}$$

17) How many mcg of dextrose are in 1 drop of 5% dextrose solution if there are 20 drops/mL?

$$1 \text{ gtt}\left(\frac{1 \text{ mL}}{20 \text{ gtts}}\right)\left(\frac{5 \text{ g}}{100 \text{ mL}}\right)\left(\frac{1,000,000 \text{ mcg}}{\text{g}}\right) = 2500 \text{ mcg}$$

18) How many g of NaCl are in 1.75 L of NS (normal saline-0.9% NaCl)?

$$1.75 \text{ L}\left(\frac{0.9 \text{ g}}{100 \text{ mL}}\right)\left(\frac{1000 \text{ mL}}{\text{L}}\right) = 15.75 \text{ g}$$

19) How many mcg of fluocinolone are in 50 g of 0.01% fluocinolone cream?

$$50 \text{ g Cr}\left(\frac{0.01 \text{ g AI}}{100 \text{ g Cr}}\right)\left(\frac{1,000,000 \text{ mcg AI}}{1 \text{ g AI}}\right) = 5000 \text{ mcg AI}$$

20) How many mg of NaCl are in 50 mL of 0.9% NaCl (normal saline)?

$$50 \text{ mL}\left(\frac{0.9 \text{ g}}{100 \text{ mL}}\right)\left(\frac{1000 \text{ mg}}{\text{g}}\right) = 450 \text{ mg}$$

Chapter 29
Percent Change Exercise

Calculate the percent change in the following scenarios. Round to the nearest tenth percent.

1) You had to adjust an IV drip from 36 gtts/min to 40 gtts/min.

$$\frac{40-36}{36}(100\%) = \frac{4}{36}(100\%) = 11.1\%$$

2) Your patient weighed 184 lb on admission and weighs 180 lb today.

$$\frac{180-184}{184}(100\%) = \frac{-4}{184}(100\%) = -2.2\%$$

3) A patient's daily dose of a drug was reduced from 50 mg to 40 mg.

$$\frac{40-50}{50}(100\%) = \frac{-10}{50}(100\%) = -20\%$$

4) A patient weighed 77 kg on Monday and still weighs 77 kg on Thursday.

$$\frac{77-77}{77}(100\%) = \frac{0}{77}(100\%) = 0\%$$

5) You increase an IV flow rate from 10.5 mL/h to 13 mL/h.

$$\frac{13-10.5}{10.5}(100\%) = \frac{2.5}{10.5}(100\%) = 23.8\%$$

6) The number of donuts in the breakroom decreased from 6 to 1 (the one nobody wants).

$$\frac{1-6}{6}(100\%) = \frac{-5}{6}(100\%) = -83.3\%$$

7) Your patient weighed 85 kg on admission and weighs 82 kg today.

$$\frac{82-85}{85}(100\%) = \frac{-3}{85}(100\%) = -3.5\%$$

8) You got a merit raise from $46.45/h to $48.05/h.

$$\frac{48.05-46.45}{46.45}(100\%) = \frac{1.60}{46.45}(100\%) = 3.4\%$$

9) The number of patients in your unit increased from 8 to 12.

$$\frac{12-8}{8}(100\%) = \frac{4}{8}(100\%) = 50\%$$

10) Your patient, who you encouraged to exercise and watch his diet, weighed 215 lb one month ago and now weighs 204 lb.

$$\frac{204-215}{215}(100\%) = \frac{-11}{215}(100\%) = -5.1\%$$

11) A dosage increased from 15 mg b.i.d to 20 mg b.i.d.

$$\frac{20-15}{15}(100\%) = \frac{5}{15}(100\%) = 33.3\%$$

12) You start a diet and reduce your caloric intake from 4500 kcal/day to 2500 kcal/day.

$$\frac{2500-4500}{4500}(100\%) = \frac{-2000}{4500}(100\%) = -44.4\%$$

13) You can now do 25 pushups but a month ago you could only do 15.

$$\frac{25-15}{15}(100\%) = \frac{10}{15}(100\%) = 66.7\%$$

14) A patient had his atorvastatin dosage lowered from 80 mg once daily to 40 mg once daily.

$$\frac{40-80}{80}(100\%) = \frac{-40}{80}(100\%) = -50\%$$

15) You increased a Pitocin drip from 2 milliunits/minute to 3 milliunits/minute.

$$\frac{3-2}{2}(100\%) = \frac{1}{2}(100\%) = 50\%$$

Chapter 30
Ratio Strength Exercise

1) How many grams of active ingredient are in 350 g of a 1:50 w/w preparation?

$$350 \text{ g prep} \left(\frac{1 \text{ g AI}}{50 \text{ g prep}}\right) = 7 \text{ g AI}$$

2) You have a 100 mL vial which is labeled 1:1000. How many mg are in 60 mL of the solution?

$$60 \text{ mL} \left(\frac{1 \text{ g}}{1000 \text{ mL}}\right) \left(\frac{1000 \text{ mg}}{\text{g}}\right) = 60 \text{ mg}$$

3) How many mcg are in 120 mL of a 1:100,000 solution?

$$120 \text{ mL} \left(\frac{1 \text{ g}}{100,000 \text{ mL}}\right) \left(\frac{1,000,000 \text{ mcg}}{\text{g}}\right) = 1200 \text{ mcg}$$

4) You have a 5 mL vial which is labeled 1:10,000 and are asked to draw up 0.4 mg of drug. How many mL would you draw?

$$0.4 \text{ mg} \left(\frac{10,000 \text{ mL}}{\text{g}}\right) \left(\frac{1 \text{ g}}{1000 \text{ mg}}\right) = 4 \text{ mL}$$

5) How many mg of active ingredient are in 500 mL of a 1:10,000 solution?

$$500 \text{ mL} \left(\frac{1 \text{ g}}{10,000 \text{ mL}}\right) \left(\frac{1000 \text{ mg}}{\text{g}}\right) = 50 \text{ mg}$$

6) How many grams of active ingredient are in 50 mL of a 1:200 solution?

$$50 \text{ mL} \left(\frac{1 \text{ g}}{200 \text{ mL}}\right) = 0.25 \text{ g}$$

7) How many grams of active ingredient are in 200 mL of a 1:10,000 solution?

$$200 \text{ mL} \left(\frac{1 \text{ g}}{10,000 \text{ mL}}\right) = 0.02 \text{ g}$$

8) You have a 50 mL vial which is labeled 1:1000 and are asked to draw up 1.4 mg. How many mL would you draw?

$$1.4 \text{ mg} \left(\frac{1000 \text{ mL}}{\text{g}}\right) \left(\frac{1 \text{ g}}{1000 \text{ mg}}\right) = 1.4 \text{ mL}$$

9) You have a solution which is 1:1000 w/v. What is the percent strength?

$$\left(\frac{1 \text{ g}}{1000 \text{ mL}}\right)(100\%) = 0.1\%$$

10) What is the percent strength of a 1:100 w/v solution?

$$\left(\frac{1 \text{ g}}{100 \text{ mL}}\right)(100\%) = 1\%$$

Chapter 31
Reconstitution Calculations Exercise

1) The physician has ordered 200 mg IM of a drug which is available in 1 g vials with instructions to add 3.6 mL SW for injection for a final concentration of 250 mg/mL. How many mL will you administer?

$$200 \text{ mg}\left(\frac{1 \text{ mL}}{250 \text{ mg}}\right) = 0.8 \text{ mL}$$

2) The physician has ordered 400 mg IM of a drug which is available in a 1000 mg vial with directions to add 4.3 mL SW for injection for a final concentration of 200 mg/mL. How many mL will you administer?

$$400 \text{ mg}\left(\frac{1 \text{ mL}}{200 \text{ mg}}\right) = 2 \text{ mL}$$

3) You have an order for 500 mg IV of a drug which is available in 1 g vials with directions to reconstitute with 8.5 mL of SW for injection for a final concentration of 100 mg/mL. How many mL will you administer?

$$500 \text{ mg}\left(\frac{1 \text{ mL}}{100 \text{ mg}}\right) = 5 \text{ mL}$$

4) A 1,000,000-unit vial of penicillin G potassium has instructions which state to reconstitute to a concentration of 100,000 units per mL, add 10 mL SW for injection. You have an order for 300,000 units IM. How many mL will you administer?

$$300,000 \text{ units}\left(\frac{1 \text{ mL}}{100,000 \text{ units}}\right) = 3 \text{ mL}$$

5) A 2 g vial states to add 7.4 mL of SW for injection for a final concentration of 200 mg/mL. You have an order for 250 mg IV. How many mL will you administer?

$$250 \text{ mg}\left(\frac{1 \text{ mL}}{200 \text{ mg}}\right) = 1.25 \text{ mL rounded to } 1.3 \text{ mL}$$

6) A 61 kg male patient diagnosed with herpes simplex encephalitis is to receive acyclovir 10 mg/kg IV infused over 1 hour, every 8 hours for 10 days. You have on hand a 1000 mg vial with the instructions to dissolve the contents of the vial in 20 mL of SWFI with the resulting solution containing 50 mg of acyclovir per mL. The calculated dose will then be withdrawn and added to a 100 mL bag of D5W. After reconstitution, what volume of the 50 mg/mL solution will you add to the 100 mL bag?

$$\left(\frac{10 \text{ mg}}{\text{kg}}\right)\left(\frac{61 \text{ kg}}{1}\right)\left(\frac{1 \text{ mL}}{50 \text{ mg}}\right) = 12.2 \text{ mL}$$

7) You are reconstituting a 150 mL bottle of amoxicillin 250 mg/5 mL. The instructions for reconstitution are as follows. Total amount of water required for reconstitution is 111 mL. Tap the bottle until all powder flows freely. Add approximately 1/3 of the total amount of water for reconstitution and shake vigorously to wet the powder. Add the remainder of the water and again shake vigorously. How many doses are contained in the bottle if the child were to take 6 mL PO t.i.d.?

$$150 \text{ mL}\left(\frac{1 \text{ dose}}{6 \text{ mL}}\right) = 25 \text{ doses}$$

8) A patient has an order for azithromycin 500 mg IV administered over 60 minutes at a concentration of 1 mg/mL. The 500 mg vial states: Prepare the initial solution of azithromycin for injection by adding 4.8 mL of Sterile Water For Injection to the vial and shaking the vial until all of the drug is dissolved. Each mL of the solution contains 100 mg of azithromycin.

a) The 5 mL vial will now be added to what size bag of NS to achieve a 1 mg/mL concentration?

$$500 \text{ mg} \left(\frac{1 \text{ mL}}{1 \text{ mg}}\right) = 500 \text{ mL}$$

Note: The small volume of 5 mL can be disregarded when added to 500 mL.

b) At what rate will you set the IV infusion pump to the nearest tenth mL/h?

$$\frac{500 \text{ mL}}{60 \text{ min}} \left(\frac{60 \text{ min}}{h}\right) = \frac{500 \text{ mL}}{h}$$

9) A patient has an order for streptomycin 500 mg IM which is available in 1 g vials with instructions to add 3.2 mL of Water for Injection USP for a final concentration of 250 mg/mL. How many mL will you administer?

$$500 \text{ mg} \left(\frac{1 \text{ mL}}{250 \text{ mg}}\right) = 2 \text{ mL}$$

10) You have an order for 350 mg IM of a drug which is available in a 500 mg vial with instructions to add 4.4 mL of SW for injection for a final concentration of 100 mg/mL. How many mL will you administer?

$$350 \text{ mg} \left(\frac{1 \text{ mL}}{100 \text{ mg}}\right) = 3.5 \text{ mL}$$

Chapter 32
Concentrations and Dilutions Exercise

1) An order calls for 600 mL of a 15% solution. You have a 40% solution on hand. How many mL of stock solution (40%) and how many mL of diluent are needed?

Using V1C1=V2C2, V1=600 mL, C1=15%, V2=unknown stock volume, C2=40%

You can either leave the percents as is or change them to decimals. For these exercises, they will be changed to decimals.

600 mL (0.15) = V2 (0.40)

V2= (600 mL x 0.15)/0.40

V2= 225 mL (stock volume)

Total volume – stock volume = diluent volume

600 mL – 225 mL = 375 mL diluent

Answer: 225 mL stock solution, 375 mL diluent

2) You have on hand a 35% stock solution. A doctor writes an order for 60 mL of a 25% solution. How many mL of the stock solution and how many mL of diluent are needed?

60 mL (0.25) = V2 (0.35)

V2= 42.9 mL (stock volume)

60 mL – 42.9 mL = 17.1 mL diluent

Answer: 42.9 mL stock solution, 17.1 mL diluent

3) An order is written for 300 mL of a 7.5% solution. You have a 50% solution available. How many mL of the stock solution and how many mL of diluent are needed?

300 mL (0.075) = V2 (0.50)

V2= 45 mL (stock volume)

300 mL – 45 mL = 255 mL diluent

Answer: 45 mL stock solution, 225 mL diluent

4) You have an order for 100 mL of a 50 mg/mL solution. Your stock bottle is labeled 300 mg/2 mL. How many mL of the stock solution and how many mL of diluent are needed?

100 mL (50 mg/mL) = V2 (300 mg/2 mL)

V2 = 100 mL (50 mg/mL) (2 mL/300 mg)

V2 = 33.3 mL (stock volume)

100 mL – 33.3 mL = 66.7 mL diluent

Answer: 33.3 mL stock solution, 66.7 mL diluent

5) The provider has ordered 3/4 strength tube-feeding formula for your patient. You have available a 240 mL container. How much water will you add to the 240 mL to prepare the 3/4 strength formula?

Using V1C1=V2C2, V1=240 mL, C1=100%, V2=unknown volume of final product, C2=75%

240 mL (1.00) = V2 (0.75)

V2= (240 mL x 1.00)/0.75

V2= 320 mL (volume of 3/4 strength formula)

Total volume – stock volume = diluent volume

320 mL – 240 mL = 80 mL water

Answer: 80 mL

Alternate method:

Let x = total volume of 3/4 strength formula

0.75x will equal the 240 mL of full-strength formula

0.75x = 240 mL

x = 320 mL

320 mL – 240 mL = 80 mL (of water)

6) The pharmacy stocks a 15% and a 75% solution. You receive an order for 300 mL of a 35% solution, but the pharmacy is too busy to help you. How many milliliters of the 15% and 75% solutions are needed?

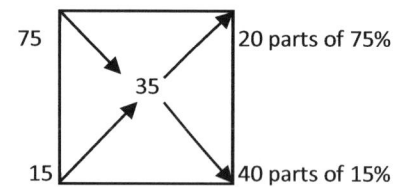

```
75                  20 parts of 75%
         35
15                  40 parts of 15%
```

The total parts are 60 (20 + 40). 20 parts out of 60 parts are 75% solution. 40 parts out of 60 are 15% solution.

$$(300 \text{ mL})\frac{20}{60} = 100 \text{ mL of } 75\%$$

$$(300 \text{ mL})\frac{40}{60} = 200 \text{ mL of } 15\%$$

7) An order is written for 500 mL of a 34% solution. Your pharmacy stocks a 10% and a 45% solution. How many milliliters of the 10% and 45% solutions are needed?

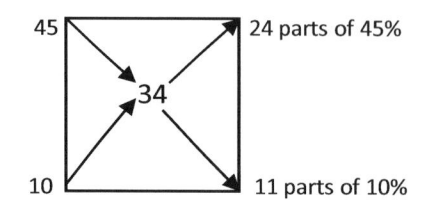

```
45                  24 parts of 45%
         34
10                  11 parts of 10%
```

The total parts are 35 (24 + 11). 24 parts out of 35 parts are 45% solution. 11 parts out of 35 parts are 10% solution.

$$(500 \text{ mL}) \frac{24}{35} = 342.9 \text{ mL of } 45\%$$

$$(500 \text{ mL}) \frac{11}{35} = 157.1 \text{ mL of } 10\%$$

8) What is the percentage strength of a mixture containing 80 mL of a 10% solution and 180 mL of a 35% solution?

$$80 \text{ mL} \left(\frac{10 \text{ g}}{100 \text{ mL}}\right) = 8 \text{ g}$$

$$180 \text{ mL} \left(\frac{35 \text{ g}}{100 \text{ mL}}\right) = 63 \text{ g}$$

The total volume is 260 mL (80 mL + 180 mL). The total weigh of active ingredient is 71 g (8 g + 63 g). (71 g/260 mL) 100% = 27.3%

9) The provider has ordered 1/2 strength tube-feeding formula for your patient. You have available a 240 mL container. How much water will you add to the 240 mL to prepare the 1/2 strength formula?

Using V1C1=V2C2, V1=240 mL, C1=100%, V2=unknown volume of final product, C2=50%

240 mL (1.00) = V2 (0.50)

V2= (240 mL x 1.00)/0.50

V2= 480 mL (volume of 1/2 strength formula)

Total volume – stock volume = diluent volume

480 mL – 240 mL = 240 mL water

Answer: 240 mL

(You should be able to do this without all the math.)

10) What is the percent strength of a mixture containing 100 mL of a 7% solution, 200 mL of a 10% solution and 700 mL of a 15% solution, all the same active ingredient?

$$100 \text{ mL} \left(\frac{7 \text{ g}}{100 \text{ mL}}\right) = 7 \text{ g}$$

$$200 \text{ mL} \left(\frac{10 \text{ g}}{100 \text{ mL}}\right) = 20 \text{ g}$$

$$700 \text{ mL} \left(\frac{15 \text{ g}}{100 \text{ mL}}\right) = 105 \text{ g}$$

The total volume is 1000 mL (100 mL + 200 mL + 700 mL). The total weigh of active ingredient is 132 g (7 g + 20 g + 105 g). (132 g/1000 mL) 100% = 13.2%

Chapter 33
Milliequivalent Calculations Exercise

1) Look up the atomic masses (atomic weights) of the following elements.

Name	Atomic Symbol	Atomic Mass (rounded to nearest tenth)	Ionic Form
Hydrogen	H	1.0	H$^+$ (Hydrogen Ion)
Carbon	C	12.0	
Oxygen	O	16.0	
Sodium	Na	23.0	Na$^+$ (Sodium Ion)
Magnesium	Mg	24.3	Mg^{++} (Magnesium Ion)
Chlorine	Cl	35.5	Cl$^-$ (Chloride Ion)
Potassium	K	39.1	K$^+$ (Potassium Ion)
Calcium	Ca	40.1	Ca^{++} (Calcium Ion)
Sulfur	S	32.1	

2) Now that you know the atomic masses of each of the elements, fill in the formula masses of the listed polyatomic ions (ions with more than one atom). Add up all the individual masses. CH$_3$COO$^-$ has two carbons atoms, three hydrogen atoms, and two oxygen atoms.

Name	Chemical Formula	Formula Mass	Ionic Form
Acetate	CH$_3$COO$^-$	59.0	CH$_3$COO$^-$
Bicarbonate	HCO$_3$-	61.0	HCO$_3^-$
Sulfate	SO$_4^{-2}$	96.1	SO$_4^{2-}$

3) List the formula masses of the following ionic compounds.

Name	Chemical Formula	Formula Mass	Ionic Form
Sodium Chloride	NaCl	58.5	Na$^+$ Cl$^-$
Potassium Chloride	KCl	74.6	K$^+$ Cl$^-$
Calcium Chloride	CaCl$_2$	111.1	Ca^{++} 2Cl$^-$
Magnesium Chloride	MgCl$_2$	95.3	Mg^{++} 2Cl$^-$
Sodium Acetate	CH$_3$COONa	82.0	Na$^+$ CH$_3$COO$^-$
Potassium Acetate	CH$_3$COOK	98.1	K$^+$ CH$_3$COO$^-$
Magnesium Sulfate	MgSO$_4$	120.4	Mg^{++} SO$_4^{2-}$
Sodium Bicarbonate	NaHCO$_3$	84.0	Na$^+$ HCO$_3^-$

4) Fill in the table with the ratios of mg/mmol and mEq/mmol for each compound.

Name	Chemical Formula	mg/mmol (ratio)	mEq/mmol (ratio)
Sodium Chloride	NaCl	58.5 mg/mmol	1 mEq/mmol
Potassium Chloride	KCl	74.6 mg/mmol	1 mEq/mmol
Calcium Chloride	CaCl$_2$	111.1 mg/mmol	2 mEq/mmol
Magnesium Chloride	MgCl$_2$	95.3 mg/mmol	2 mEq/mmol
Sodium Acetate	CH$_3$COONa	82.0 mg/mmol	1 mEq/mmol
Potassium Acetate	CH$_3$COOK	98.1 mg/mmol	1 mEq/mmol
Magnesium Sulfate	MgSO$_4$	120.4 mg/mmol	2 mEq/mmol
Sodium Bicarbonate	NaHCO$_3$	84.0 mg/mmol	1 mEq/mmol

5) How many mEq of MgSO₄ are contained in 13 g of MgSO₄?

$$13\text{ g}\left(\frac{1\text{ mmol}}{120.4\text{ mg}}\right)\left(\frac{2\text{ mEq}}{\text{mmol}}\right)\left(\frac{1000\text{ mg}}{\text{g}}\right) = 215.9\text{ mEq}$$

6) How many mEq of NaCl are in 2 L of 0.45% NaCl?

$$2\text{ L}\left(\frac{0.45\text{ g}}{100\text{ mL}}\right)\left(\frac{1000\text{ mL}}{\text{L}}\right)\left(\frac{1000\text{ mg}}{\text{g}}\right)\left(\frac{1\text{ mmol}}{58.5\text{ mg}}\right)\left(\frac{1\text{ mEq}}{\text{mmol}}\right) = 153.8\text{ mEq}$$

7) How many mEq of calcium chloride are contained in 2.5 g of calcium chloride?

$$2.5\text{ g}\left(\frac{1\text{ mmol}}{111.1\text{ mg}}\right)\left(\frac{2\text{ mEq}}{\text{mmol}}\right)\left(\frac{1000\text{ mg}}{\text{g}}\right) = 45\text{ mEq}$$

8) How many mEq of Ca⁺⁺ are in 1.4 g of calcium chloride?

$$1.4\text{ g}\left(\frac{1\text{ mmol}}{111.1\text{ mg}}\right)\left(\frac{2\text{ mEq}}{\text{mmol}}\right)\left(\frac{1000\text{ mg}}{\text{g}}\right) = 25.2\text{ mEq}$$

9) How many mEq of K⁺ are contained in 250 mg of KCl?

$$250\text{ mg}\left(\frac{1\text{ mmol}}{74.6\text{ mg}}\right)\left(\frac{1\text{ mEq}}{\text{mmol}}\right) = 3.4\text{ mEq}$$

10) How many grams of Na⁺ (just the sodium) are contained in 3.5 L of 10% NaCl?

$$3.5\text{ L}\left(\frac{10\text{ g NaCl}}{100\text{ mL}}\right)\left(\frac{1000\text{ mL}}{\text{L}}\right)\left(\frac{23\text{ g Na}^+}{58.5\text{ g NaCl}}\right) = 137.6\text{ g Na}^+$$

11) How many mg of magnesium sulfate are in 40 mEq of magnesium sulfate?

$$40\text{ mEq}\left(\frac{1\text{ mmol}}{2\text{ mEq}}\right)\left(\frac{120.4\text{ mg}}{\text{mmol}}\right) = 2408\text{ mg}$$

12) How many mEq of KCl are in 20 mL of 10% KCl solution?

$$20\text{ mL}\left(\frac{10\text{ g}}{100\text{ mL}}\right)\left(\frac{1000\text{ mg}}{\text{g}}\right)\left(\frac{1\text{ mmol}}{74.6\text{ mg}}\right)\left(\frac{1\text{ mEq}}{\text{mmol}}\right) = 26.8\text{ mEq}$$

13) How many g of sodium acetate are in 25 mEq of sodium acetate?

$$25\text{ mEq}\left(\frac{1\text{ mmol}}{1\text{ mEq}}\right)\left(\frac{82\text{ mg}}{\text{mmol}}\right)\left(\frac{1\text{ g}}{1000\text{ mg}}\right) = 2.1\text{ g}$$

14) How many mg of KCl are in 60 mL of 2 mEq/mL KCl?

$$60\text{ mL}\left(\frac{2\text{ mEq}}{\text{mL}}\right)\left(\frac{74.6\text{ mg}}{\text{mmol}}\right)\left(\frac{1\text{ mmol}}{\text{mEq}}\right) = 8952\text{ mg}$$

Chapter 34
Dosage Calculation Puzzles

1) You have an order to start an IV infusion at x mL/h, where 3x + 25= 175, on your patient Mr. Whipple, who is recovering from wrist surgery. The IV bag contains y mg/ z mL, where 3y + z = 620 and y-z = -460. Mr. Whipple weighs 73 kg. How many mcg/kg/min is Mr. receiving?

Step 1) Solve for x, y and z.

3x + 25 = 175

3x = 150

x = 50

3y + z = 620

z = 620 − 3y

y − (620 − 3y) = -460

y − 620 + 3y = -460

4y = 160

y = 40

40 − z = -460

-z = -500

z = 500

Step 2)

Infusion rate = 50 mL/h

IV bag contains 40 mg/500 mL

Step 3) Set up and solve equation.

$$\frac{50 \text{ mL}}{\text{h}} \left(\frac{1 \text{ h}}{60 \text{ min}}\right)\left(\frac{40 \text{ mg}}{500 \text{ mL}}\right)\left(\frac{1}{73 \text{ kg}}\right)\left(\frac{1000 \text{ mcg}}{\text{mg}}\right) = \frac{0.91 \text{ mcg}}{\text{kg min}}$$

Answer: 0.91 mcg/kg/min

2) You have an order for 1 g of a drug to infuse over 4 hours. The pharmacy sends you a 1 L bag labeled: contains 250 mL of 3 mg/mL, 250 mL of 2 mg/mL, 250 mL of 5 mg/mL and 250 mL of NS.

a) At what rate will you set the pump?

Step 1) Calculate total volume and mg of drug in the bag.

$$250 \text{ mL} \left(\frac{3 \text{ mg}}{\text{mL}}\right) = 750 \text{ mg}$$

$$250 \text{ mL} \left(\frac{2 \text{ mg}}{\text{mL}}\right) = 500 \text{ mg}$$

$$250 \text{ mL} \left(\frac{5 \text{ mg}}{\text{mL}}\right) = 1250 \text{ mg}$$

$$250 \text{ mL} \left(\frac{0 \text{ mg}}{\text{mL}}\right) = 0 \text{ mg}$$

Total mg = 2500 mg Total volume = 1000 mL

2500 mg/1000 mL

Step 2) Calculate volume of solution which contains 1 g.

$$1 \text{ g} \left(\frac{1000 \text{ mL}}{2500 \text{ mg}}\right) \left(\frac{1000 \text{ mg}}{\text{g}}\right) = 400 \text{ mL}$$

You will infuse 400 mL over 4 h.

$$\frac{400 \text{ mL}}{4 \text{ h}} = \frac{100 \text{ mL}}{\text{h}}$$

Answer: 100 mL/h

b) You started the infusion at 1300. You check on the patient at 1400 only to learn that the patient turned off the pump at 1345 because his friend told him that he didn't need any big pharma drugs. After explaining the importance of the drug to the patient, you get out your calculator and note pad. At what rate will you set the pump to finish the 1 g infusion on time if you restart the infusion at 1415?

At 1345 the pump had been running for 45 minutes. 45 min (100 mL/60 min) = 75 mL infused, leaving 325 mL to be infused. At 1415 you would have 2 h 45 minutes remaining until 1700, which is when the infusion was scheduled to end.

$$\frac{325 \text{ mL}}{2.75 \text{ h}} = \frac{118.2 \text{ mL}}{\text{h}}$$

Answer: 118.2 mL/h

3) A new miracle drug is released by the FDA which reverses aging by 25% in adults over 50 YO. The dosage is 3 mg/kg + 2.5 mg for each year over 50 years old, rounded to the nearest 10 mg, given IV over 2 hours. The drug is available in 25 mg vials with instructions to reconstitute each vial with 8 mL of supplied diluent to yield a concentration of 2.5 mg/mL. Your facility's protocol is to reconstitute the appropriate number of vials and add to a 500 mL bag of D5W after withdrawing an equal volume of reconstituted drug from the 500 mL bag, then infuse over 2 hours. The drug, Youngme, is very expensive at $250/mg. Your facility has a new policy stating that the nurse who administers the drug must also calculate the charge of the drug and collect the cash payment. Your patient, Mr. Wrinkles, is 74 years old and weighs 80 kg. He is a little concerned about the price of the drug and relays to you that he makes $23.50/hour as a professional dog food taster. Mr. Wrinkles works 8 hours/day, five days per week. What will be the total charge for Mr. Wrinkles' therapy and how many weeks, days and hours will he have to work to pay for it?

Step 1) Calculate the dose in mg Mr. Wrinkles will require.

$$\frac{3 \text{ mg}}{\text{kg}} \left(\frac{80 \text{ kg}}{1}\right) = 240 \text{ mg}$$

74 years – 50 years = 24 years over 50 years old

$$24 \text{ years} \left(\frac{2.5 \text{ mg}}{\text{year}}\right) = 60 \text{ mg}$$

Total dose = 300 mg

Step 2) Calculate the cost of the 300 mg

$$300 \text{ mg} \left(\frac{\$250}{\text{mg}}\right) = \$75,000$$

Step 3) Calculate number of hours Mr. Wrinkles must work at $23.50/h to pay for the treatment.

$$\$75,000 \left(\frac{1 \text{ h}}{\$23.50}\right) = 3191.49 \text{ h rounded to } 3191 \text{ h}$$

Step 4) Convert 3191 h to weeks.

$$3191 \text{ h} \left(\frac{1 \text{ week}}{40 \text{ h}}\right) = 79.775 \text{ weeks}$$

Step 5) Convert 0.775 weeks to days at 5 days/week.

$$0.775 \text{ week} \left(\frac{5 \text{ days}}{\text{week}}\right) = 3.875 \text{ days}$$

Step 6) Convert 0.875 days to hours at 8 h/day.

$$0.875 \text{ day} \left(\frac{8 \text{ h}}{\text{day}}\right) = 7 \text{ h}$$

Step 7) Add up the weeks, days and hours.

Answer: 79 weeks, 3 days, 7 hours

Chapter 35
Self-Assessment Exam

The exam has 100 questions, each worth one point.

Convert the following:

1) 60 mL = L   60 mL (1 L/1000 mL) = **0.06 L**

2) 4.5 g = mg   4.5 g (1000 mg/g) = **4500 mg**

3) 2 tbs = mL   2 tbs (15 mL/tbss) = **30 mL**

4) 1.5 cups = mL   1.5 cups (240 mL/cup) = **360 mL**

5) 120 mL = fl oz   120 mL (1 fl oz/30 mL) = **4 fl oz**

6) 178 lb = kg   178 lb (1 kg/2.2 lb) = **80.9 kg**

7) 8.5 cm = in   8.5 cm (1 in/2.54 cm) = **3.3 in**

8) 1.85 kg = lb   1.85 kg (2.2 lb/kg) = **4.1 lb**

9) 140 g = kg   140 g (1 kg/1000 g) = **0.14 kg**

10) 3 tbs = mL   3 tbs (15 mL/tbs) = **45 mL**

Round the following numbers to the nearest tenth.

11) 6.43   **6.4**

12) 0.186   **0.2**

13) 5.96   **6.0**

14) 0.0005   **0.0**

15) 38.044   **38.0**

Round the following numbers to the nearest hundredth.

16) 16.874   **16.87**

17) 4.047   **4.05**

18) 31.006   **31.01**

19) 0.0565   **0.06**

20) 4.168   **4.17**

Write the corresponding Roman numerals for the following numbers:

21) 9   **IX**

22) 4   **IV**

23) 22   **XXII**

24) 43   **XLIII**

25) 125   **CXXV**

Dosage Calculations for Nursing Students-Second Edition

Write the corresponding numbers for the following Roman numerals:

26) VIII   **8**

27) LIX   **59**

28) XXXII   **32**

29) CXI   **111**

30) CX   **110**

Convert the following to scientific notation:

31) 320,000 3.2×10^5

32) 162,000,000 1.62×10^8

33) 0.0000054 5.4×10^{-6}

34) 45,000 4.5×10^4

35) 249,000 2.49×10^5

Convert the following from scientific notation to numbers.

36) 8.34×10^5 **834,000**

37) 9.202×10^5 **920,200**

38) 2.302×10^{-6} **0.000002302**

39) 5.15×10^{-8} **0.0000000515**

40) 6.104×10^7 **61,040,000**

Answer the following questions concerning military time.

41) You started studying for your exam at 1700 and finished at 2230. How many hours and minutes did you study?

5 h 30 min

42) What is 4:25 PM in military time?

1625

43) You start and IV at 0800 which is scheduled to run 8 hours. What time will it end in military time?

1600

44) A patient is to receive a medication every 8 hours around the clock. He received doses at 0600 and 1400. When should he receive the next dose?

2200

45) You are asked to work from 10:00 AM to 1800. Your employer tells you that you can either be paid $37.50 per hour or a flat rate of $325. Which is the better deal for you?

$325 is the better deal.

Dosage Calculations for Nursing Students-Second Edition

Convert the following numbers to percents.

46) 0.06   **0.06 (100%) = 6%**

47) 1.35   **1.35 (100%) = 135%**

48) 0.475   **0.475 (100%) = 47.5%**

Convert the following percents to numbers.

49) 83.1%   **83.1%/100% = 0.831**

50) 100%   **100%/100% = 1**

51) 0.152%   **0.152%/100% = 0.00152**

Express the following as percent strength solutions and include the type of solution (w/w, w/v, v/v, v/w).

52) 7.5 g NaCl in 1000 mL   **(7.5 g/1000 mL) (100%) = 0.75% w/v**

53) 1.6 g KCl in 100 mL   **(1.6 g/100 mL) (100%) = 1.6% w/v**

54) 40 mL ETOH in 160 mL.   **(40 mL ETOH/160 mL)(100%) = 25% v/v**

Answer the following:

55) How many mg of lidocaine are in 250 mL of 1% lidocaine solution?

$$250 \text{ mL} \left(\frac{1 \text{ g}}{100 \text{ mL}}\right)\left(\frac{1000 \text{ mg}}{\text{g}}\right) = 2500 \text{ mg}$$

56) How many mg of triamcinolone are in 45 g of 0.5% triamcinolone cream?

$$45 \text{ g cr} \left(\frac{0.5 \text{ g AI}}{100 \text{ g cr}}\right)\left(\frac{1000 \text{ mg AI}}{\text{g cr}}\right) = 225 \text{ mg AI}$$

57) How many mg of NaCl are in 400 mL of 0.9% NaCl?

$$400 \text{ mL} \left(\frac{0.9 \text{ g}}{100 \text{ mL}}\right)\left(\frac{1000 \text{ mg}}{\text{g}}\right) = 3600 \text{ mg}$$

Answer the following questions pertaining to percent change.

58) You weigh 162 lb on August 1st and spend the next week hiking around Yosemite National Park. On August 8th you weigh 152 lb. What is the percent change in your weight?

$$\frac{152 - 162}{162}(100\%) = \frac{-10}{162}(100\%) = -6.2\%$$

59) You have two hamsters who fall in love and have 4 babies. What is the percent change in your hamster population?

$$\frac{6 - 2}{2}(100\%) = \frac{4}{2}(100\%) = 200\%$$

60) The physician changed a patient's dose of a drug from 50 mg to 25 mg. What is the percent change in the dose?

$$\frac{25 - 50}{50}(100\%) = \frac{-25}{50}(100\%) = -50\%$$

61) Kristina F, a nursing student, scored 80% on her dosage calculation quiz on Monday. The following Monday she scored 98%. What is the percent change in her grade?

$$\frac{98-80}{80}(100\%) = \frac{18}{80}(100\%) = 22.5\%$$

62) Your patient weighed 75 kg on admission and now weighs 73 kg. What is the percent change in the patient's weight?

$$\frac{73-75}{75}(100\%) = \frac{-2}{75}(100\%) = -2.7\%$$

Answer the following dosage questions.

63) The PCP has ordered 80 mg IM of a drug which is available in 200 mg/mL. How many mL will you administer?

$$80 \text{ mg}\left(\frac{1 \text{ mL}}{200 \text{ mg}}\right) = 0.4 \text{ mL}$$

64) The physician has ordered 40 mg IV of a drug which is available in 5 mL vials of 10 mg/mL. How many mL will you administer?

$$40 \text{ mg}\left(\frac{1 \text{ mL}}{10 \text{ mg}}\right) = 4 \text{ mL}$$

65) The NP ordered 80 mg PO once daily for a patient. The drug is available in 40 mg tablets. How many tablets will the patient take each day?

$$80 \text{ mg}\left(\frac{1 \text{ tab}}{40 \text{ mg}}\right) = 2 \text{ tabs}$$

66) The physician has ordered 90 mg IM of a drug which is available in 10 mL vials containing 45 mg/mL. How many mL will you administer?

$$90 \text{ mg}\left(\frac{1 \text{ mL}}{45 \text{ mg}}\right) = 2 \text{ mL}$$

67) Your patient has an order for 12.5 mg PO of a drug which is available in 5 mg scored tablets. How many tabs will you administer?

$$12.5 \text{ mg}\left(\frac{1 \text{ tab}}{5 \text{ mg}}\right) = 2.5 \text{ tabs}$$

68) Your 52 YO patient, who weighs 165 lb, has an order for drug xyz 100 mg/day divided into two doses. Drug xyz is available in 10 mL vials containing 40 mg/mL. How many mL will you administer per dose?

$$\frac{100 \text{ mg}}{\text{day}}\left(\frac{1 \text{ day}}{2 \text{ doses}}\right)\left(\frac{1 \text{ mL}}{40 \text{ mg}}\right) = \frac{1.25 \text{ mL}}{\text{dose}} \text{ rounded to } \frac{1.3 \text{ mL}}{\text{dose}}$$

69) You have an order to administer 100 mcg/day PO divided into two doses. You have 0.025 mg tablets available. How many tablets will you administer per dose?

$$\frac{100 \text{ mcg}}{\text{day}}\left(\frac{1 \text{ day}}{2 \text{ doses}}\right)\left(\frac{1 \text{ tab}}{0.025 \text{ mg}}\right)\left(\frac{1 \text{ mg}}{1000 \text{ mcg}}\right) = \frac{2 \text{ tabs}}{\text{dose}}$$

70) Your patient has an order for 250 mg IV every 6 hours of a drug which is available in 10 mL vials containing 25 mg/mL. How many mL will be administered in 24 hours?

$$\frac{250 \text{ mg}}{\text{dose}}\left(\frac{4 \text{ doses}}{\text{day}}\right)\left(\frac{1 \text{ mL}}{25 \text{ mg}}\right) = \frac{40 \text{ mL}}{\text{day}}$$

71) The physician has ordered 500 mcg IM of a drug which is available in 2 mL vials containing 0.5 mg/mL. How many mL will you administer?

$$500 \text{ mcg} \left(\frac{1 \text{ mL}}{0.5 \text{ mg}}\right)\left(\frac{1 \text{ mg}}{1000 \text{ mcg}}\right) = 1 \text{ mL}$$

72) The physician has ordered 60 mg IV of a drug which is available in 5 mL vials containing 20 mg/mL. How many mL will you administer?

$$60 \text{ mg} \left(\frac{1 \text{ mL}}{20 \text{ mg}}\right) = 3 \text{ mL}$$

73) A 39 lb child has an order for furosemide 2 mg/kg PO once daily. Furosemide oral solution is available in 60 mL bottles containing 10 mg/mL. How many mL will you administer per dose?

$$\frac{2 \text{ mg}}{\text{kg}} \left(\frac{39 \text{ lb}}{1}\right)\left(\frac{1 \text{ kg}}{2.2 \text{ lb}}\right)\left(\frac{1 \text{ mL}}{10 \text{ mg}}\right) = 3.5 \text{ mL}$$

74) A 78 kg patient is to receive an initial bolus dose of a drug 0.085 mg/kg over at least 2 minutes. The drug is available in 4 mL vials containing 2.5 mg/mL. How many mL will you administer?

$$\frac{0.085 \text{ mg}}{\text{kg}} \left(\frac{78 \text{ kg}}{1}\right)\left(\frac{1 \text{ mL}}{2.5 \text{ mg}}\right) = 2.7 \text{ mL}$$

75) A 155 lb patient is to receive a single IV dose of ondansetron 0.15 mg/kg for prevention of nausea and vomiting. Ondansetron is available in 20 mL MDV of 2 mg/mL. How many mL will you administer?

$$\frac{0.15 \text{ mg}}{\text{kg}} \left(\frac{155 \text{ lb}}{1}\right)\left(\frac{1 \text{ kg}}{2.2 \text{ lb}}\right)\left(\frac{1 \text{ mL}}{2 \text{ mg}}\right) = 5.3 \text{ mL}$$

Calculate the flow rate in mL per hour rounded to the nearest tenth mL/h.

76) 1000 mL infused over 8 hours.

$$\frac{1000 \text{ mL}}{8 \text{ h}} = \frac{125 \text{ mL}}{\text{h}}$$

77) 500 mL infused over 7 hours.

$$\frac{500 \text{ mL}}{7 \text{ h}} = \frac{71.4 \text{ mL}}{\text{h}}$$

78) 1000 mL infused over 6 hours.

$$\frac{1000 \text{ mL}}{6 \text{ h}} = \frac{166.7 \text{ mL}}{\text{h}}$$

79) 100 mL infused over 30 minutes.

$$\frac{100 \text{ mL}}{0.5 \text{ h}} = \frac{200 \text{ mL}}{\text{h}}$$

Calculate the flow rate in drops/min. Round to the nearest whole drop.

80) 500 mL infused over 6 hours with a drop factor of 20 (20 gtts/mL).

$$\frac{500 \text{ mL}}{6 \text{ h}} \left(\frac{1 \text{ h}}{60 \text{ min}}\right)\left(\frac{20 \text{ gtts}}{\text{mL}}\right) = \frac{28 \text{ gtts}}{\text{min}}$$

81) 1000 mL infused over 5 hours with a drop factor of 10.

$$\frac{1000 \text{ mL}}{5 \text{ h}}\left(\frac{1 \text{ h}}{60 \text{ min}}\right)\left(\frac{10 \text{ gtts}}{\text{mL}}\right) = \frac{33 \text{ gtts}}{\text{min}}$$

82) 250 mL infused over 3 hours with a drop factor of 15.

$$\frac{250 \text{ mL}}{3 \text{ h}}\left(\frac{1 \text{ h}}{60 \text{ min}}\right)\left(\frac{15 \text{ gtts}}{\text{mL}}\right) = \frac{21 \text{ gtts}}{\text{min}}$$

83) 500 mL infused over 8 hours with a microdrip set (60 gtts/mL).

$$\frac{500 \text{ mL}}{8 \text{ h}}\left(\frac{1 \text{ h}}{60 \text{ min}}\right)\left(\frac{60 \text{ gtts}}{\text{mL}}\right) = \frac{63 \text{ gtts}}{\text{min}}$$

Calculate the length of time in hours and minutes, rounded to the nearest minute, required to infuse the following:

84) 500 mL at 45 mL/h.

$$500 \text{ mL}\left(\frac{1 \text{ h}}{45 \text{ mL}}\right) = 11.11 \text{ h} = 11 \text{ h } 7 \text{ min}$$

85) 750 mL at 90 mL/h.

$$750 \text{ mL}\left(\frac{1 \text{ h}}{90 \text{ mL}}\right) = 8.33 \text{ h} = 8 \text{ h } 20 \text{ min}$$

86) 500 mL at 55 gtts/min with a drop factor of 20.

$$500 \text{ mL}\left(\frac{1 \text{ min}}{55 \text{ gtts}}\right)\left(\frac{20 \text{ gtts}}{\text{mL}}\right) = 182 \text{ min} = 3 \text{ h } 2 \text{ min}$$

87) 1 L at 36 gtts/min with a drop factor of 15.

$$1 \text{ L}\left(\frac{1000 \text{ mL}}{\text{L}}\right)\left(\frac{1 \text{ min}}{36 \text{ gtts}}\right)\left(\frac{15 \text{ gtts}}{\text{mL}}\right) = 417 \text{ min} = 6 \text{ h } 57 \text{ min}$$

Calculate the volume infused in the following scenarios.

88) Infusion rate of 30 mL/h for 5 h 30 min.

$$5.5 \text{ h}\left(\frac{30 \text{ mL}}{\text{h}}\right) = 165 \text{ mL}$$

89) Infusion rate of 28 gtts/min, drop factor 20, for 3 hours 45 min.

$$3.75 \text{ h}\left(\frac{28 \text{ gtts}}{\text{min}}\right)\left(\frac{1 \text{ mL}}{20 \text{ gtts}}\right)\left(\frac{60 \text{ min}}{\text{h}}\right) = 315 \text{ mL}$$

Calculate the following. Round all drops/min to the nearest drop and all mL/h rates to the nearest tenth mL/h.

90) Your 61 kg patient has an order for a lidocaine infusion at the rate of 20 mcg/kg/min. You have a 250 mL bag labeled "Lidocaine HCl and 5% Dextrose Injection USP". Lidocaine 2 g (8 mg/mL) is printed in big red letters in the middle of the label. What rate will you set the IV infusion pump?

$$\frac{20 \text{ mcg}}{\text{kg min}}\left(\frac{61 \text{ kg}}{1}\right)\left(\frac{1 \text{ mL}}{8 \text{ mg}}\right)\left(\frac{1 \text{ mg}}{1000 \text{ mcg}}\right)\left(\frac{60 \text{ min}}{\text{h}}\right) = \frac{9.2 \text{ mL}}{\text{h}}$$

91) Your 160 lb patient, who has been diagnosed with septic shock, has an order for norepinephrine 0.15 mcg/kg/min IV. The pharmacy delivers a bag containing 4 mg norepinephrine in 250 mL D5NS. At what rate will you set the IV infusion pump?

$$\frac{0.15 \text{ mcg}}{\text{kg min}}\left(\frac{160 \text{ lb}}{1}\right)\left(\frac{1 \text{ kg}}{2.2 \text{ lb}}\right)\left(\frac{250 \text{ mL}}{4 \text{ mg}}\right)\left(\frac{1 \text{ mg}}{1000 \text{ mcg}}\right)\left(\frac{60 \text{ min}}{\text{h}}\right) = \frac{40.9 \text{ mL}}{\text{h}}$$

92) Your 172 lb female patient has an order for dobutamine 5 mcg/kg/min IV to start at 1300. The dobutamine is available as 1000 mcg/mL. At what rate will you set the IV infusion pump?

$$\frac{5 \text{ mcg}}{\text{kg min}}\left(\frac{172 \text{ lb}}{1}\right)\left(\frac{1 \text{ kg}}{2.2 \text{ lb}}\right)\left(\frac{1 \text{ mL}}{1000 \text{ mcg}}\right)\left(\frac{60 \text{ min}}{\text{h}}\right) = \frac{23.5 \text{ mL}}{\text{h}}$$

Answer the following reconstitution calculation questions.

93) You have an order for 150 mg IM of a drug which is available in 1 g vials with directions to reconstitute with 8.5 mL of SW for injection for a final concentration of 100 mg/mL. How many mL will you administer?

$$150 \text{ mg}\left(\frac{1 \text{ mL}}{100 \text{ mg}}\right) = 1.5 \text{ mL}$$

94) A patient has an order for 500 mg IM of a drug which is available in 1 g vials with instructions to add 3.2 mL of Water for Injection USP for a final concentration of 250 mg/mL. How many mL will you administer?

$$500 \text{ mg}\left(\frac{1 \text{ mL}}{250 \text{ mg}}\right) = 2 \text{ mL}$$

Calculate the BSA in m² for the following people using the Mosteller formula.

95) An adult male weighing 175 lb and 5 ft 11 in tall.

$$\sqrt{\frac{175 \times 71}{3131}} = 1.99 \text{ m}^2$$

96) A 14-month-old girl weighing 22 lb and 30 in tall.

$$\sqrt{\frac{22 \times 30}{3131}} = 0.46 \text{ m}^2$$

97) An adult male weighing 93 kg and 185 cm tall.

$$\sqrt{\frac{93 \times 185}{3600}} = 2.19 \text{ m}^2$$

Answer the following:

98) The provider ordered 3/4 strength formula tube feeding for your patient. How much water would you add to a 180 mL container of full-strength formula?

V1C1=V2C2

180 mL (100%) = V2 (75%)

V2=240 mL (total volume of ¾ strength formula)

240 mL – 180 mL = 60 mL

Answer: 60 mL water

99) A mEq of Na⁺ and a mEq of K⁺ weigh the same. T or F

False

100) A mEq of Na⁺ and a mEq of K⁺ contain the same number of ions. T or F

True

Printed in Great Britain
by Amazon